Autism and Child Psychopathology Series

Series Editor
Johnny L. Matson
Department of Psychology
Louisiana State University
Baton Rouge, LA, USA

For further volumes:
http://www.springer.com/series/8665

Jennifer B. Ganz

Aided Augmentative Communication for Individuals with Autism Spectrum Disorders

With contributions by
Ee Rea Hong and Whitney Gilliland

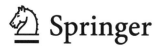 Springer

6719

KH

Jennifer B. Ganz
Texas A&M University
College Station, TX, USA

ISSN 2192-922X ISSN 2192-9238 (electronic)
ISBN 978-1-4939-5338-7 ISBN 978-1-4939-0814-1 (eBook)
DOI 10.1007/978-1-4939-0814-1
Springer New York Heidelberg Dordrecht London

2|10|20

Preface

This book is the sum of the past 18 years of my professional career. When I was a special education teacher, I worked with young children across a broad range of the autism spectrum – from students with social and behavioral issues who spoke fluently to those with "classic autism" traits who could neither speak nor write in a manner that was understandable. I was and am most drawn to these children, for whom it seemed needed a key or an "a-ha" moment to unlock effective communication. I attended all the training opportunities I could and apprenticed under my more experienced colleagues to learn how to best teach these children. For children who could not speak, it became clear to me that aided augmentative and alternative communication (AAC) could be that key. However, I met with much resistance from some of my students' parents who were afraid that aided AAC would give their children an easy way out of having to talk. Unfortunately, at that time, there was little research to support the idea that aided AAC could serve as an effective means of providing the ability to communicate to children with autism and that it would not inhibit speech. Yet, my, albeit limited, experiences had convinced me that this could serve as a way for these children to communicate and that, for some children, the concrete nature of AAC may provide a link to unlocking speech and understanding of communication in general. Thus, I embarked on graduate school and then my career in academia, where I have tried to determine the impacts of AAC on people with autism and synthesize the body of literature in this area. Although much research has been published by myself and many others, and many types of aided AAC have come to be recognized, I believe there is much work left to do. This book is my attempt to further pull together the state of the art and to suggest where the field should go from here.

College Station, TX, USA   Jennifer B. Ganz

Contents

About the Author

Jennifer B. Ganz, Ph.D., BC.B.A-.D. conducts research on high- and low-tech interventions to improve social and communication skills in individuals with autism spectrum disorders and other developmental disabilities, with a particular focus on augmentative and alternative communication and autism. She has two decades of experience with people with developmental and other disabilities as a researcher, presenter, consultant, special education teacher, and general education teacher. Dr. Ganz is currently a Professor of special education at Texas A&M University.

Contributors

Ee Rea Hong is a doctoral candidate in special education at Texas A&M University and is a Board Certified Behavior Analyst. Her research interests are related to individuals with autism spectrum disorders and development of their language and communication skills. In particular, Ee Rea Hong is passionate about conducting research to help to teach and support families of individuals with autism.

Whitney Gilliland's research focus is on transition/post-secondary issues for people with autism spectrum disorders, particularly improvement of employment skills. She is currently a doctoral student in special education at Texas A&M University.

Part I
Introduction and Overview

Chapter 1
Overview of Autism Spectrum Disorders and Complex Communication Needs

Current estimates suggest that approximately 1 in 68 children has an autism spectrum disorder (ASD; Centers for Disease Control and Prevention [CDC] 2014). Further, over one million children in the USA have complex communication needs (CCN), meaning that they cannot effectively use speech to communicate (Binger and Light 2006). Many people with ASD have CCN as well. Recognizing that an individual with ASD has significant problems communicating well through speech is critical to ensuring that these communication needs are addressed early to prevent a loss of educational and social opportunities (Horovitz and Matson 2010). Thus, this chapter provides readers with a brief overview of characteristics of ASD, with a significant focus on people with ASD who also have CCN, laying the groundwork for later chapters that address what can and should be done to address significant communication needs in this population.

Characteristics of ASDs

ASDs fall across a broad spectrum. That is, people who have ASD are a heterogeneous group. The range of functioning and skills may fall at any point on a wide scale. The key characteristics that qualify someone for a diagnosis of an ASD are observable deficits in social–communication skills and the presence of restrictive, repetitive, and stereotypical interests and/or behaviors. Each of these areas, and other deficit and skill areas that are common in individuals with ASD, is discussed below, with a focus on the subgroup of individuals with ASD for whom augmentative and alternative communication (AAC) may be most appropriate.

The diagnostic criteria for ASD in the Diagnostic and Statistical Manual (DSM-5; American Psychiatric Association [APA] 2013), which is the primary tool for diagnosing ASD in the USA, have been modified significantly from the prior edition.

J.B. Ganz, *Aided Augmentative Communication for Individuals with Autism Spectrum Disorders*, Autism and Child Psychopathology Series, DOI 10.1007/978-1-4939-0814-1_1,
© Springer Science+Business Media New York 2014

Major changes include the combination of the social and communication factors into a single category. To qualify as having an ASD, the DSM-5 states that individuals must meet the three social–communication criteria and at least two of the four criteria related to restricted and repetitive behaviors. Further, in the DSM-5, subcategories of ASD [e.g., pervasive developmental disorder, not otherwise specified (PDD-NOS)] have been replaced with a spectrum model involving severity in social communication and in restricted/repetitive behaviors (APA 2013). Individuals who meet the criteria for ASD are now further categorized as having or not having a language impairment; that is, previously, one of the possible qualifying criteria was a lack of functional speech, or the preverbal communication phase (Tager-Flusberg et al. 2009), which instead is now considered an "add on" specification and would be considered as likely qualifying an individual as having a "level 3" severity for social communication, or "requiring very substantial supports" (APA 2013).

The DSM-5 (APA 2013) changes have caused some concern that the criteria are now more strict and will eliminate people with mild ASD and young children who do not immediately demonstrate enough of the social–communication deficits due to age, decreasing the probability of early intervention (Barton et al. 2013). In fact, a number of recent studies have reported that, under the new criteria, many high functioning individuals of all ages, people with PDD-NOS, those with fewer challenging behaviors, and young children with ASD would no longer qualify (Barton et al. 2013; Gibbs et al. 2012; Mandy et al. 2012; Matson et al. 2012a, b; McPartland et al. 2012; Volkmar and Reichow 2013; Williams et al. 2013; Wilson et al. 2013). It has also been suggested that young children who previously met the criteria, but would no longer under the current edition, have significant impairments when compared to typically developing peers, particularly in expressive communication (Beighley et al. 2014). Researchers have recommended that the DSM-5 ASD criteria be adjusted to improve sensitivity (i.e., reduction of false negatives, or failure to diagnose a child with ASD who does have it) and specificity (i.e., reduction in false positive diagnoses) by reducing the number of social-communication and restricted and repetitive behaviors criteria necessary for a diagnosis (Frazier et al. 2012; Kent et al. 2013; Lohr and Tanguay 2013).

Social–Communication Skills

Social and communication differences often become more apparent as people with ASD age and social interactions and expectations become more complex (Tantam 2003). To qualify as having ASD, the individual being evaluated must have the following three characteristics in social interaction and communication (APA 2013). First, he or she must have deficits in emotional reciprocity. For example, people with ASD typically have difficulties understanding and perceiving others' feelings and thoughts (Kuo et al. 2013). They may be less oriented toward other people than their peers are, such that the quality and quantity of their interactions may appear significantly different (Kuo et al. 2013). Children with ASD often have less awareness of the need to share interests and take turns (Rowley et al. 2012).

Second, he or she must have difficulty appropriately using and interpreting non-verbal communication (APA 2013). For example, people with ASD may have difficulty interpreting facial expressions or combining messages given through tone of voice, body posture, and facial expression, causing incorrect interpretations. People with ASD are likely to avoid making eye contact to the degree others do (Matson et al. 2009b). Some speak in monotone or have unusual pitch or use of stresses in speech (Kanner 1971). Further, it may be difficult for them to match tone and facial expressions to emotions (Shriberg et al. 2001).

Third, he or she must have difficulties forming and sustaining relationships with others to a significant degree. For example, people with ASD often have difficulty demonstrating interest in others and maintaining contact to a degree expected by others their age (APA 2013). Although many do report that they have some friends (Kuo et al. 2013), they have fewer friendships and are more likely to have no friends than peers (Rowley et al. 2012). Their perceptions of friendships tend to indicate less intimacy or closeness than their peers do in relationships with other typically developing peers (Solomon et al. 2011). Further, adolescents with ASD have been found to spend more time with paid professionals and other adults and to socialize with adults more than their peers do (Orsmond and Kou 2011; Solish et al. 2010). Adolescents with ASD also report fewer opposite-gender friends than do their peers, which could lead to less likelihood of romantic relationships (Kuo et al. 2013). Relatedly, students with ASD are more frequently the targets of bullying than peers with other disabilities (Humphrey and Symes 2010) and typically developing peers (Rowley et al. 2012). Frequently people with ASD prefer to be alone when compared to people with intellectual disabilities who do not have ASD (Matson et al. 2009b). Play deficits are common in younger children with ASD (Barrett et al. 2004).

ASD and CCN. Although severe speech deficits are no longer among the defining criteria for ASD (APA 2013), people with ASD have a wide range of language abilities, from those who are able to use complex and fluent sentences to those who cannot speak (Matson et al. 2010b; Grzadzinski et al. 2013). Humans use language to fulfill varied purposes, including interacting socially, communicating needs, protesting, and learning (Sigafoos et al. 2006); the lack of ability to effectively communicate may negatively impact communicative, social, behavioral, and academic outcomes (Branson and Demchak 2009), particularly post-secondary outcomes (Hamm and Mirenda 2006). Individuals with ASD who require adult services are particularly unlikely to use speech as a primary means of communicating; that is, approximately half of adults receiving developmental disability services use speech as a primary means of communication (Hewitt et al. 2012). Further, ASD with CCN is often associated with intellectual disabilities (Luyster et al. 2008) and oral-motor difficulties (Gernsbacher et al. 2008). Thus, those who have ASD and CCN require special considerations when developing interventions, particularly AAC interventions.

Restrictive, Repetitive, and Stereotypical Interests and Behaviors

According to the current DSM-5 (APA 2013), to qualify as having an ASD, in addition to the abovementioned social–communication deficits, the individual must meet at least two of the following four criteria. One, he or she may engage in speech or motor movements that are repetitive or stereotyped (APA 2013). This can include unusual motor movements, seeking sensory stimulation, and using items in a repetitive, typically not functional, manner (Cuccaro et al. 2003). Repetitive motor movements are particularly common in younger children with ASD and those with more significant intellectual impairments (Fombonne 2003), while repetitive speech is more common in people with ASD who are older and have higher intellectual functioning (Bishop et al. 2006).

Two, he or she may be particularly drawn to routines and rituals involving verbal and/or nonverbal behaviors or be particularly resistant to change (APA 2013). For example, people with ASD may display compulsive behavior related to repetitive routines and display challenging behavior or otherwise resist change in routines or the environment (Cuccaro et al. 2003). Insistence on sameness has been demonstrated to be linked to structural brain differences (Bishop et al. 2013).

Three, he or she may have intensely focused restricted interests compared to others (APA 2013). For instance, a person with ASD may have a strong interest in automatic sprinkler systems and repetitively discuss types of systems and accessories in great detail. This characteristic is more common in people with ASD who are older and higher functioning (Bishop et al. 2006; Carcani-Rathwell et al. 2006). Four, he or she may be over- or under-sensitive to sensory stimuli or be intensely interested in sensory stimuli (APA 2013). For example, he or she might sniff people's hair or flick lights on and off.

Challenging Behaviors and ASD

Although challenging behavior, or behavior that is problematic given a particular context [i.e., socially unacceptable, harmful, and reduces quality of life (Matson et al. 2010a)], is not a core or defining characteristic of ASD (DSM citation), individuals with ASD often display such difficulties (Hill and Furniss 2006; Mandy et al. 2012). More specifically, some people with ASD have been described as engaging in tantrums, aggressive, oppositional, and noncompliant behaviors (Kaat and Lecavalier 2013) and have been found to engage in such behaviors more often than typically developing peers and peers with other disabilities such as attention deficit hyperactivity disorder (Konst et al. 2013; Mayes et al. 2012). Some people with ASD engage in self-injurious behaviors, such as banging their heads against hard surfaces or biting themselves (Katt and Lecavalier). Challenging behaviors tend to be more severe in individuals with more significant intellectual impairments (Gray et al. 2012). With age, however, behaviors tend to improve for most people with ASD, although for individuals with severe intellectual disabilities, behaviors tend to increase (Gray et al. 2012).

It is thought that individuals with ASD often engage in challenging behavior to communicate needs, particularly when they cannot effectively communicate verbally (Chiang 2008; Kaat and Lecavalier 2013). People with ASD and CCN may resort to challenging behaviors (e.g., self-injurious behaviors, aggression, property damage) if unable to effectively communicate (Ganz et al. 2009). Research has revealed that people with ASD frequently engage in challenging behaviors to communicate a desire to escape demands or gain access to preferred items and activities, including those related to their preferred repetitive motor movements (Matson et al. 2011; Reese et al. 2005). Further, more severe communication and social skill deficits are associated with higher rates of challenging behavior (Konst et al. 2013; Matson et al. 2009a; Sigafoos 2000) and higher rates of restricted and repetitive behaviors (Ray-Subramanian and Ellis Weismer 2012). Thus, providing people with ASD and CCN with a reliable means of communicating may address challenging behaviors while addressing communication deficits.

Commonly Co-occurring Conditions and Characteristics

Often, ASD is diagnosed concomitantly with other disabilities, and features of ASD are similar to characteristics of some other disabilities. For example, individuals with deafblindness and significant intellectual impairments have similar impairments in communication and social interaction, as well as stereotypy (Hoevenaars-van den Boom et al. 2009). Characteristics prevalent in people with ASD have been found to be more common in people with Down syndrome (Moss et al. 2013) and Prader-Willi syndrome than in the general population (Buono et al. 2010).

Further, people with ASD are at an increased risk of having a number of co-occurring disabilities. High rates of psychiatric diagnoses have been found in adolescents and adults with ASD (Mandy et al. 2014). For example, people with ASD have been diagnosed with attention deficit hyperactivity disorder, anxiety disorder, and oppositional defiant disorder at higher rates than found in the general population (Gadow et al. 2005; Mandy et al. 2012; Simonoff et al. 2008; Ung et al. 2013). An estimated 25–40 % of children with ASD meet the diagnostic criteria for either conduct disorder or oppositional defiant disorder (Kaat and Lecavalier 2013; Mayes et al. 2012). Symptoms of depression are common in people with ASD, particularly those who are higher functioning (Sterling et al. 2008). Approximately 38 % of children with ASD have IQs in the range of intellectual disability ($\leq$70; CDC 2014), which is correlated with a higher risk for lacking the ability to speak (Hewitt et al. 2012).

Augmentative and Alternative Communication

The purpose of AAC is to improve the communicative competence of people who have CCN (Light 1997a, b; Lund and Light 2006). In a nutshell, communicative competence for people who use AAC involves improving the quality and quantity of communicative interactions in daily life, not in clinical treatment settings (Light 1989, 1997a; Sutton 1989; Teachman and Gibson 2014). As noted above, AAC may provide a socially acceptable means for individuals with ASD and CCN to communicate, resulting in a decrease in the need to engage in challenging behaviors along with enhanced communication and interaction (Ganz et al. 2009). Further, aided AAC, or high- or low-tech devices such as picture communication boards and computerized devices, is thought to be well suited to individuals with ASD because it is primarily visually based, provides concrete representations of abstract concepts, does not require advanced motor skills, and serves as a tool through which people with CCN can communicate and engage in social activities (Cafiero and Meyer 2008). The remaining chapters in this book will provide suggestions for practitioners and parents regarding assessment for and selection of aided AAC systems, collaborating with others to implement AAC, AAC-based interventions, and controversial issues related to AAC for people with ASD and CCN.

References

American Psychiatric Association (APA). (2013). *Diagnostic and statistical manual* (5th ed.). Washington, DC: American Psychiatric Association (APA).

Barrett, S., Prior, M., & Manjiviona, J. (2004). Children on the borderlands of autism: Differential characteristics in social, imaginative, communicative and repetitive behaviour domains. *Autism, 8*, 61–87. doi:10.1177/1362361304040640.

Barton, M. L., Robins, D. L., Jashar, D., Brennan, L., & Fein, D. (2013). Sensitivity and specificity of proposed DSM-5 criteria for autism spectrum disorder in toddlers. *Journal of Autism and Developmental Disorders, 43*, 1184–1195. doi:10.1007/s10803-013-1817-8.

Beighley, J. S., Matson, J. L., Rieske, R. D., Konst, M. J., & Tureck, K. (2014). Differences in communication skills in toddlers diagnosed with autism spectrum disorder according to the DSM-IV-TR and the DSM-5. *Research in Autism Spectrum Disorders, 8*, 74–81. doi:10.1016/j.rasd.2013.10.014.

Binger, C., & Light, J. (2006). Demographics of preschoolers who require AAC. *Language, Speech, and Hearing Services in Schools, 37*, 200–208.

Bishop, S. L., Hus, V., Duncan, A., Huerta, M., Gotham, K., Pickles, A., & Lord, C. (2013). Subcategories of restricted and repetitive behaviors in children with autism spectrum disorders. *Journal of Autism and Developmental Disorders, 43*, 1287–1297. doi:10.1007/s10803-012-1671-0.

Bishop, S. L., Richler, J., & Lord, C. (2006). Association between restricted and repetitive behaviors and nonverbal IQ in children with autism spectrum disorders. *Child Neuropsychology, 12*, 247–267.

Branson, D., & Demchak, M. (2009). The use of augmentative and alternative communication methods with infants and toddlers with disabilities: A research review. *Augmentative and Alternative Communication, 25*, 274–286.

Buono, S., Scannella, F., & Palmigiano, M. B. (2010). Self-injurious behavior: A comparison between Prader-Willi syndrome, Down syndrome and autism. *Life Span and Disability, 13*, 187–201.

Cafiero, J. M., & Meyer, A. (2008). Your child with autism: When is augmentative and alternative communication (AAC) an appropriate option? *Exceptional Parent, 38*, 28–30.

Carcani-Rathwell, I., Rabe-Hasketh, S., & Santosh, P. J. (2006). Repetitive and stereotyped behaviours in pervasive developmental disorders. *Journal of Child Psychology and Psychiatry, 47*, 573–581. doi:10.1111/j.1469-7610.2005.01565.x.

Centers for Disease Control and Prevention. (2014). Prevalence of autism spectrum disorders among children aged 8 years—Autism and developmental disabilities monitoring network, 11 sites, United States, 2010. *Morbidity and Mortality Weekly Report, 63*(SS-3), 1–21.

Chiang, H. (2008). Expressive communication of children with autism: The use of challenging behaviour. *Journal of Intellectual Disability Research, 52,* 966–972. doi:10.1111/j.1365-2788.2008.01042.x.

Cuccaro, M. L., Shao, Y., Grubber, J., Slifer, M., Wolpert, C. M., Donnelly, S. L., … Pericak-Vance, M. A. (2003). Factor analysis of restricted and repetitive behaviors in autism using the Autism Diagnostic Interview-R. *Child Psychiatry and Human Development, 34*(1), 3–17.

Fombonne, E. (2003). Epidemiological surveys of autism and other pervasive developmental disorders: An update. *Journal of Autism and Developmental Disorders, 33,* 365–381.

Frazier, T. W., Youngstrom, E. A., Speer, L., Embacher, R., Law, P., Constantino, J., … Eng, C. (2012). Validation of proposed DSM-5 criteria for autism spectrum disorder. *Journal of the American Academy of Child and Adolescent Psychiatry, 51,* 28–40.e3. doi: 10.1016/j.jaac.2011.09.021

Gadow, K. D., DeVincent, C. T., Pomeroy, J., & Azizian, A. (2005). Comparison of DSM-IV symptoms in elementary school-age children with PDD versus clinical and community samples. *Autism: The International Journal of Research and Practice, 9,* 392–415.

Ganz, J. B., Parker, R., & Benson, J. (2009). Impact of the picture exchange communication system: Effects on communication and collateral effects on maladaptive behaviors. *Augmentative and Alternative Communication, 25,* 250–261. doi:10.3109/07434610903381111.

Gernsbacher, M., Sauer, E., Geye, H., Schweigert, E., & Goldsmith, H. (2008). Infant and toddler oral- and manual-motor skills predict later speech fluency in autism. *Journal of Child Psychology and Psychiatry, 49,* 43–50.

Gibbs, V., Aldridge, F., Chandler, F., Witzlsperger, E., & Smith, K. (2012). Brief report: An exploratory study comparing diagnostic outcomes for autism spectrum disorders under DSM-IV-TR with the proposed DSM-5 revision. *Journal of Autism and Developmental Disorders, 42,* 1750–1756. doi:10.1007/s10803-012-1560-6.

Gray, K., Keating, C., Taffe, J., Brereton, A., Einfeld, S., & Tonge, B. (2012). Trajectory of behavior and emotional problems in autism. *American Journal on Intellectual and Developmental Disabilities, 117,* 121–133. doi:10.1352/1944-7588-117-2.121.

Grzadzinski, R., Huerta, M., & Lord, C. (2013). DSM-5 and autism spectrum disorders (ASDs): An opportunity for identifying ASD subtypes. *Molecular Autism, 4*(12), 1–6. doi:10.1186/2040-2392-4-12.

Hamm, B., & Mirenda, P. (2006). Post-school quality of life for individuals with developmental disabilities who use AAC. *Augmentative and Alternative Communication, 22,* 134–147. doi:10.1080/07434610500395493.

Hewitt, A. S., Stancliffe, R. J., Johnson Sirek, A., Hall-Lande, J., Taub, S., Engler, J., & Moseley, C. R. (2012). Characteristics of adults with autism spectrum disorder who use adult developmental disability services: Results from 25 US states. *Research in Autism Spectrum Disorders, 6,* 741–751. doi:10.1016/j.rasd.2011.10.007.

Hill, J., & Furniss, F. (2006). Patterns of emotional and behavioral disturbance associated with autistic traits in young people with severe intellectual disabilities and challenging behaviors. *Research in Developmental Disabilities, 27,* 517–528.

Hoevenaars-van den Boom, M. A. A., Antonissen, A. C. F. M., Knoors, H., & Vervloed, M. P. J. (2009). Differentiating characteristics of deafblindness and autism in people with congenital deafblindness and profound intellectual disability. *Journal of Intellectual Disability Research, 53,* 548–558. doi:10.1111/j.1365-2788.2009.01175.x.

Horovitz, M., & Matson, J. L. (2010). Communication deficits in babies and infants with autism and pervasive developmental disorder-not otherwise specified (PDD-NOS). *Developmental Neurorehabilitation, 13,* 390–398.

Humphrey, N., & Symes, W. (2010). Perceptions of social support and experience of bullying among pupils with autistic spectrum disorders in mainstream secondary schools. *European Journal of Special Needs Educational, 25,* 77–91.

Kaat, A. J., & Lecavalier, L. (2013). Disruptive behavior disorders in children and adolescents with autism spectrum disorders: A review of the prevalence, presentation, and treatment. *Research in Autism Spectrum Disorders, 7*, 1579–1594. doi:10.1016/j.rasd.2013.08.012.

Kanner, L. (1971). Follow-up of eleven autistic children, originally reported in 1943. *Journal of Autism and Childhood Schizophrenia, 2*, 119–145.

Kent, R. G., Carrington, S. J., Le Couteur, A., Gould, J., Wing, L., Maljaars, J., & Leekam, S. R. (2013). Diagnosing autism spectrum disorder: Who will get a DSM-5 diagnosis? *Journal of Child Psychology and Psychiatry, and Allied Disciplines, 54*, 1242–1250. doi:10.1111/jcpp.12085.

Konst, M. J., Matson, J. L., & Turygin, N. (2013). Exploration of the correlation between autism spectrum disorder symptomology and tantrum behaviors. *Research in Autism Spectrum Disorders, 7*, 1068–1074. doi:10.1016/j.rasd.2013.05.006.

Kuo, M. H., Orsmond, G. I., Cohn, E. S., & Coster, W. J. (2013). Friendship characteristics and activity patterns of adolescents with an autism spectrum disorder. *Autism, 17*, 481–500. doi:10.1177/1362361311416380.

Light, J. (1989). Toward a definition of communicative competence for individuals using augmentative and alternative communication systems. *Augmentative and Alternative Communication, 5*, 137–144. doi:10.1080/07434618912331275126.

Light, J. (1997a). "Communication is the essence of human life": Reflections on communicative competence. *Augmentative and Alternative Communication, 13*, 61–70.

Light, J. (1997b). "Let's go star fishing": Reflections on the contexts of language learning for children who use aided AAC. *Augmentative and Alternative Communication, 13*, 158–171. doi:10.1080/07434619712331277978.

Lohr, W. D., & Tanguay, P. (2013). DSM-5 and proposed changes to the diagnosis of autism. *Pediatric Annals, 42*, 161–166. doi:10.3928/00904481-20130326-12.

Lund, S., & Light, J. (2006). Long-term outcomes for individuals who use augmentative and alternative communication: Part I—what is a "good" outcome? *Augmentative and Alternative Communication, 22*, 284–299.

Luyster, R., Kadlec, M., Carter, A., & Tager-Flusberg, H. (2008). Language assessment and development in toddlers with autism spectrum disorders. *Journal of Autism and Developmental Disorders, 38*, 1426–1438.

Mandy, W. P., Charman, T., & Skuse, D. H. (2012). Testing the construct validity of proposed criteria for DSM5 autism spectrum disorder. *Journal of the American Academy of Child and Adolescent Psychiatry, 51*, 41–50.

Mandy, W., Roughan, L., & Skuse, D. (2014). Three dimensions of oppositionality in autism spectrum disorder. *Journal of Abnormal Child Psychology, 42*, 291–300. doi: 10.1007/s10802-013-9778-0

Matson, J. L., Belva, B. C., Horovitz, M., Kozlowski, A. M., & Bamburg, J. W. (2012a). Comparing symptoms of autism spectrum disorders in a developmentally disabled adult population using the current DSM-IV-TR diagnostic criteria and the proposed DSM-5 diagnostic criteria. *Journal of Developmental and Physical Disabilities, 24*, 403–414. doi:10.1007/s10882-012-9278-0.

Matson, J. L., Boisjoli, J., & Mahan, S. (2009a). The relation of communication and challenging behaviors in infants and toddlers with autism spectrum disorders. *Journal of Developmental and Physical Disabilities, 21*, 253–261. doi:10.1007/s10882-009-9140-1.

Matson, J. L., Dempsey, T., & LoVullo, S. V. (2009b). Characteristics of social skills for adults with intellectual disability, autism and PDD-NOS. *Research in Autism Spectrum Disorders, 3*, 207–213. doi:10.1016/j.rasd.2008.05.006.

Matson, J. L., Kozlowski, A. M., Hattier, M. A., Horovitz, M., & Sipes, M. (2012b). DSM-IV vs DSM-5 diagnostic criteria for toddlers with autism. *Developmental Neurorehabilitation, 15*, 185–190. doi:10.3109/17518423.2012.672341.

Matson, J. L., Mahan, S., Hess, J., Fodstad, J. C., & Neal, D. (2010a). Progression of challenging behaviors in children and adolescents with autism spectrum disorders as measured by the Autism Spectrum Disorder—Problem Behaviors For Children (ASD-PBC). *Research in Autism Spectrum Disorders, 4*, 400–404.

Matson, J. L., Mahan, S., Kozlowski, A. M., & Shoemaker, M. (2010b). Developmental milestones in toddlers with autistic disorder, pervasive developmental disorder-not otherwise specified and atypical development. *Developmental Neurorehabilitation, 13*, 239–247. doi:10.3109/1751842 3.2010.481299.

Matson, J. L., Sipes, M., Horovitz, M., Worley, J. A., Shoemaker, M. E., & Kozlowski, A. M. (2011). Behaviors and corresponding functions addressed via functional assessment. *Research in Developmental Disabilities, 32*, 625–629.

Mayes, S. D., Calhoun, S. L., Aggarwal, R., Baker, C., Mathapati, S., Anderson, R., & Petersen, C. (2012). Explosive, oppositional, and aggressive behavior in children with autism compared to other clinical disorders and typical children. *Research in Autism Spectrum Disorders, 6*, 1–10. doi:10.1016/j.rasd.2011.08.001.

McPartland, J. C., Reichow, B., & Volkmar, F. R. (2012). Sensitivity and specificity of proposed DSM5 diagnostic criteria for autism spectrum disorder. *Journal of the American Academy of Child and Adolescent Psychiatry, 51*, 368–383.

Moss, J., Richards, C., Nelson, L., & Oliver, C. (2013). Prevalence of autism spectrum disorder symptomatology and related behavioural characteristics in individuals with down syndrome. *Autism, 17*, 390–404. doi:10.1177/1362361312442790.

Orsmond, G. I., & Kou, H. (2011). The daily lives of adolescents with an autism spectrum disorder: Discretionary time use and activity partners. *Autism, 15*, 1–21.

Ray-Subramanian, C. E., & Ellis Weismer, S. (2012). Receptive and expressive language as predictors of restricted and repetitive behaviors in young children with autism spectrum disorders. *Journal of Autism and Developmental Disorders, 42*, 2113–2120. doi:10.1007/s10803-012-1463-6.

Reese, R. M., Richman, D. M., Belmont, J. M., & Morse, P. (2005). Functional characteristics of disruptive behavior in developmentally delayed children with and without autism. *Journal of Autism and Developmental Disorders, 35*, 419–428.

Rowley, E., Chandler, S., Baird, G., Simonoff, E., Pickles, A., Loucas, T., & Charman, T. (2012). The experience of friendship, victimization and bullying in children with an autism spectrum disorder: Associations with child characteristics and school placement. *Research in Autism Spectrum Disorders, 6*, 1126–1134. doi:10.1016/j.rasd.2012.03.004.

Shriberg, L. D., Paul, R., McSweeny, J. L., Klin, A., Cohen, D. J., & Volkmar, F. R. (2001). Speech and prosody characteristics of adolescents and adults with high-functioning autism and Asperger syndrome. *Journal of Speech, Language, and Hearing Research, 44*, 1097–1115.

Sigafoos, J. (2000). Communication development and aberrant behavior in children with developmental disabilities. *Education and Training in Mental Retardation and Developmental Disabilities, 35*, 168–176.

Sigafoos, J., Arthur-Kelly, M., & Butterfield, N. (2006). *Enhancing everyday communication for children with disabilities*. Baltimore, MD: Paul H Brookes Publishing Co.

Simonoff, E., Pickles, A., Charman, T., Chandler, S., Loucas, T., & Baird, G. (2008). Psychiatric disorders in children with autism spectrum disorders: Prevalence, comorbidity, and associated factors in a population-derived sample. *Journal of the American Academy of Child and Adolescent Psychiatry, 47*, 9210929.

Solish, A., Perry, A., & Minnes, P. (2010). Participation of children with and without disabilities in social, recreational and leisure activities. *Journal of Applied Research in Intellectual Disabilities, 23*, 226–236.

Solomon, M., Bauminger, N., & Rogers, S. (2011). Abstract reasoning and friendship in high functioning preadolescents with autism spectrum disorders. *Journal of Autism and Developmental Disorders, 41*, 32–43.

Sterling, L., Dawson, G., Estes, A., & Greenson, J. (2008). Characteristics associated with presence of depressive symptoms in adults with autism spectrum disorder. *Journal of Autism and Developmental Disorders, 38*, 1011–1018. doi:10.1007/s10803-007-0477-y.

Sutton, A. C. (1989). The social-verbal competence of AAC users. *Augmentative and Alternative Communication, 5*, 150–164. doi:10.1080/07434618912331275156.

Tager-Flusberg, H., Rogers, S., Cooper, J., Landa, R., Lord, C., Paul, R., & Yoder, P. (2009). Defining spoken language benchmarks and selecting measures of expressive language development for young children with autism spectrum disorders. *Journal of Speech, Language, and Hearing Research, 52*, 643–652. doi:10.1044/1092-4388(2009/08-0136).

Tantam, D. (2003). The challenge of adolescents and adults with Asperger syndrome. *Child and Adolescent Psychiatric Clinics of North America, 12*, 143–163.

Teachman, G., & Gibson, B. E. (2014). 'Communicative competence' in the field of augmentative and alternative communication: A review and critique. *International Journal of Language and Communication Disorders, 49*, 1–14. doi:10.1111/1460-6984.12055.

Ung, D., Wood, J. J., Ehrenreich-May, J., Arnold, E. B., Fujii, C., Renno, P., & Storch, E. A. (2013). Clinical characteristics of high-functioning youth with autism spectrum disorder and anxiety. *Neuropsychiatry, 3*, 147–157. doi:10.2217/npy.13.9.

Volkmar, F. R., & Reichow, B. (2013). Autism in DSM-5: Progress and challenges. *Molecular Autism, 4*(13), 1–6. doi:10.1186/2040-2392-4-13.

Williams, L. W., Matson, J. L., Jang, J., Beighley, J. S., Rieske, R. D., & Adams, H. L. (2013). Challenging behaviors in toddlers diagnosed with autism spectrum disorders with the DSM-IV-TR and the proposed DSM-5 criteria. *Research in Autism Spectrum Disorders, 7*, 966–972. doi:10.1016/j.rasd.2013.03.010.

Wilson, C. E., Gillan, N., Spain, D., Robertson, D., Roberts, G., Murphy, C. M., & Murphy, D. G. M. (2013). Comparison of ICD-10R, DSM-IV-TR and DSM-5 in an adult autism spectrum disorder diagnostic clinic. *Journal of Autism and Developmental Disorders, 43*, 2515–2525. doi:10.1007/s10803-013-1799-6.

Chapter 2
Aided Augmentative and Alternative Communication: An Overview

Augmentative and alternative communication (AAC) includes any mode of expressive or receptive communication that is used to replace or supplement spoken communication for a person with a disability who cannot use conventional speech (Romski and Sevcik 1997). AAC may be unaided, such as systems that do not require external equipment, e.g., manual sign language and gestures (Light et al. 1998). Alternately, AAC can be aided. Aided AAC includes devices and external equipment such as communication boards with drawings, cards with picture or words that are exchanged, and computerized devices with or without verbal output (Light et al. 1998). Below, aided AAC will be described and research on aided AAC will be reviewed, followed by conclusions and suggestions for future research. An overview of the use of manual sign language with people with ASD and related research is provided in Chap. 9.

Aided AAC ranges from low-tech, including single pictures or icons on cards or printed arrays of drawings, to high-tech, sophisticated devices, including devices with one or more pads to select pictures and generate speech, computerized devices dedicated for communication purposes, and more recently, tablet computer and smart phone communication applications (McNaughton and Light 2013).

Low-Tech Aided AAC

Low-tech AAC has been widely used, including systems that require the person with CCN to point to pictures, letters, or words and those that involve exchanging icons, or picture cards, with someone to make a request or otherwise impart information (Ganz et al. 2012b). The pictures, words, or letters may be fixed on a single-page array or may be affixed to a book or surface by Velcro® to allow them to be taken off. Advantages of low-tech aided AAC include portability, ease of creation of new materials, low expense, low probability of loss or damage, and ease of interpretation by much of the public (Ganz et al. 2012b). Much of the literature involving low-tech AAC for people with ASD involves a well-defined system and protocol,

J.B. Ganz, *Aided Augmentative Communication for Individuals with Autism Spectrum Disorders*, Autism and Child Psychopathology Series, DOI 10.1007/978-1-4939-0814-1_2,
© Springer Science+Business Media New York 2014

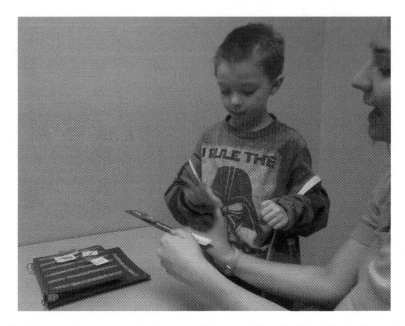

Fig. 2.1 Exchange-based communication system. Photo credit: Jennifer Ninci. Used with permission

called the Picture Exchange Communication System (PECS; Frost and Bondy 2002); other picture exchange or picture point systems are described in the literature, but are not used as widely or following a precise treatment protocol (Ganz et al. 2012b). An example of a picture exchange-based AAC book is shown in Fig. 2.1.

The Picture Exchange Communication System

Although PECS is only one type of picture-based, low-tech aided AAC, it involves a distinct instructional protocol, was developed specifically for people with ASD, and has received significant attention in the last decade (Bondy 2012; Ganz et al. 2012a); thus, it is worth describing it in detail in this chapter. PECS was developed for individuals with autism spectrum disorders and complex communication needs (Bondy 2012), that is, individuals who cannot use speech as their primary means of functionally communicating. PECS is a type of alternative and augmentative communication (AAC) system. PECS is considered a low-tech AAC system. It is made up of a binder with Velcro® strips attached and icons, or picture cards, that are stored in the binder. The icons are used by the individual with ASD to communicate. The person hands a picture or pictures to a communication partner, often an adult or peer, to make a request, comment, answer a question, or otherwise engage in conversation.

PECS was developed specifically for individuals with ASD and has been used with people with a variety of developmental disabilities. The developers, Andy Bondy and Lori Frost (1994), created the treatment protocol while working with individuals at the Delaware Autistic Program in the 1980s. The system begins with teaching requesting preferred items because children with ASD are infrequently motivated to participate in communicative interactions for purely social purposes (Bondy 2012). That is, typically developing children often use initial language skills for social means (e.g., getting attention, labeling something in the immediate environment), while children with ASD often communicate primarily to gain preferred items. Thus, Frost and Bondy (2002) suggest that beginning communication with requesting is a logical first step.

Implementation of PECS is based on applied behavior analysis (Bondy 2012). That is, discrete, evidence-based teaching procedures are used to teach new communication skills, based on Skinner's (1957) analysis of verbal and other communicative behavior. These techniques include prompting and prompt-fading (e.g., full physical prompts, partial physical prompt), backward chaining (e.g., fading prompts beginning with the final step in a chain of behaviors) (Bondy 2012). The summary of PECS instruction that follows should not be considered a replacement for attending a formal training.

PECS Phases of Instruction. There are six primary phases within the PECS protocol (Frost and Bondy 2002). Prior to instruction, a reinforcer assessment is conducted (Frost and Bondy 2002). This may be an informal assessment, involving asking caregivers to identify the client's preferred items and activities, but often also includes formally placing items in front of the client and collecting data regarding which items are picked most often (Frost and Bondy 2002). Preference assessments may be repeated, formally or informally, often, as preferred items vary over time and even within a day, depending on recent deprivation or satiation or changing desires. That is, for example, if a child has recently had 2 h of access to a favorite movie, he or she is unlikely to be motivated to request that movie.

The terminal goal in Phase 1 is that the student learns to independently pick up a picture card and hand it to a communicative partner in exchange for a preferred item, food, or activity (Frost and Bondy 2002). Instruction in Phases 1 and 2 requires two trainers. In Phase 1, one instructor sits or stands behind the learner, serving as the prompter, and the other sits or stands in front of the learner, serving as the communicative partner. The communicative partner places a picture card in front of the learner and entices the learner, such as by showing the learner a preferred item, taking a bite of a preferred food, and holding the item out toward the learner. The prompter waits for the learner to show interest or motivation to take it. The learner may do so by reaching for the object, looking at it and leaning toward it, or vocalizing. If the learner does not show interest in the item, the communicative partner exchanges the item for another preferred item and replaces the picture card with a corresponding picture card. When the learner does show interest in the item, the physical prompter, who does not engage in communication with the learner, provides a full physical prompt to assist the learner in picking up the picture card, handing it to the communicative partner, and placing it in the communicative partner's hand. These physical prompts are rapidly faded until the learner independently and spontaneously picks up the picture and places it in the communicative partner's hand in exchange for a preferred item. Key strategies during Phase 1 include backward chaining (i.e., fading prompts from the end of the sequence—placing the picture in the communicative partner's hand—to the beginning), introducing a wide variety of picture cards and corresponding items, targeting PECS instruction across a wide variety of contexts and settings, and including a variety of communicative partners. It is important in Phase 1 and throughout PECS instruction that instruction is not restricted to limited contexts or the learner may fail to generalize PECS use across contexts, materials, and communicative partners, thus, preventing it from being a truly functional communication system.

Phase 2 of PECS is an extension of Phase 1 (Frost and Bondy 2002). The learner is taught to use PECS across farther distances. That is, the terminal outcome for Phase 2 is that the learner will retrieve his or her PECS communication binder, retrieve the desired picture from the front of the book, and bring it to a communicative partner, possibly in another room. Two instructors are required in Phase 2. In initial stages, the physical prompter remains behind the learner. The learner's communication book remains within arm's reach of the learner and the communicative partner entices the learner with a preferred item while moving just out of reach. That is, the communicative partner begins Phase 2 instruction far enough away that the learner must take a step or two to place the picture card in his or her hand. The learner may independently stand and bring the picture card to the communicative partner; however, if he or she takes the card, but does not move closer, the physical prompter nudges or provides other physical prompts to assist the learner in moving toward the communicative partner. As in Phase 1, the physical prompts are quickly faded. The communicative partner gradually moves farther away, then gradually moves the communication book farther away until the learner independently exchanges pictures across a wide range of distances.

In Phase 3, the learner is taught to discriminate among pictures to select the one that corresponds with one of a variety of preferred items (Frost and Bondy 2002). By the end of Phase 3 instruction, the learner should be able to select the correct picture from among numerous placed through his or her communication book. Phase 3 and beyond do not require two instructors. Phase 3 has two stages. In Phase 3a, two picture cards are placed on the front of the communication book—one of a preferred item and one of an item that the learner does not like. As before, the communicative partner entices the learner with a preferred item. If the learner reaches for the incorrect picture, the communicative partner blocks the learner, then conducts an error correction procedure, which includes modeling the correct response by holding up the correct picture and naming it, prompting the learner to hand the correct picture by pointing to it or physically prompting, inserting a distraction by turning the book over or asking the learner to follow a quick, previously mastered task, and presenting the item again. Phase 3b involves presenting two or more pictures of preferred items, eventually leading to the child selecting from among numerous pictures within or on the cover of the communication book. Phase 3b instruction is identical to Phase 3a, with the addition of periodic correspondence checks. A correspondence check involves determining whether or not the student is accurately discriminating between the available pictures. When the student makes errors, Frost and Bondy (2002) recommend structured error-correction procedures.

In Phase 4, the client is taught to create simple sentences to make requests, combining an *I-WANT* symbol with an icon of a preferred item (Bondy 2012; Frost and Bondy 2002). The instructor uses backward chaining to first teach the client to place the preferred item's icon onto a sentence strip that already contains the *I-WANT* icon and hand the entire sentence strip to the communicative partner. Eventually, these supports are faded until the client learns to place the *I-WANT* icon and the preferred item icon on the strip and independently taking it off the book to hand to the communicative partner. Eventually, the client is taught to combine requests for multiple items into a single sentence and to add modifiers to requests (e.g., *I-WANT APPLES-TO-APPLES™ GAME*). Phases 5 and 6 involve teaching the clients to answer questions regarding what they want and see and to comment on their surrounding (Bondy 2012).

High-Tech Aided AAC

AAC technologies are rapidly becoming more portable and less expensive (Shane et al. 2012). Further, they are becoming more commonly used, via tablet computer and smartphone apps, as speech-generating devices (SGDs), along with other interventions for people with ASD and DD (Ganz et al. 2014; Kagohara et al. 2013; Murdock et al. 2013). SGDs, also sometimes called voice-output communication aids (VOCAs), have been used as AAC for several decades. Because they have natural-speech or synthesized speech output, it provides a means for the individual with CCN to get the attention of the listener and can be understood easily (Romski and Sevcik 1997; Schepis et al. 1998). These devices are electronic and range in sophistication from single buttons with recorded voice messages to small computers that allow the user and caregivers to program and add vocabulary. While low-tech systems may be either picture point or picture exchange, SGDs involve pressing, touching, or selecting a button or icon that is attached or integrated into the SGD (Shane et al. 2012; Son et al. 2006). Figures 2.2, 2.3, 2.4, 2.5, 2.6, and 2.7 provide examples of a range of low- to high-tech AAC systems.

As mobile devices have become ubiquitous in the USA (Gal et al. 2009), there has been an upsurge in studies incorporating the use of applications on table computers and smartphones for use as SGDs (Flores et al. 2012; Kagohara et al. 2013; van der Meer et al. 2012). There are numerous advantages to software and applications for mobile technologies compared to traditional SGDs that are often large and heavy, particularly considering that people with ASD, unlike people with physical

Fig. 2.2 Picture point
communication system.
Photo credit: Jennifer Ninci.
Used with permission. The
picture communication
symbols ©1981–2010 by
Mayer-Johnson LLC. All
Rights Reserved Worldwide.
Used with permission.
Boardmaker™ is a trademark
of Mayer-Johnson LLC

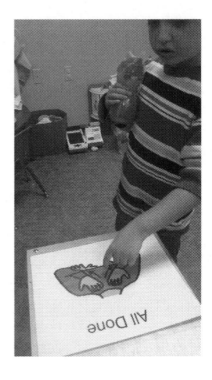

Fig. 2.3 Example of a
single-switch AAC device.
Photo credit: Jennifer Ninci.
Used with permission

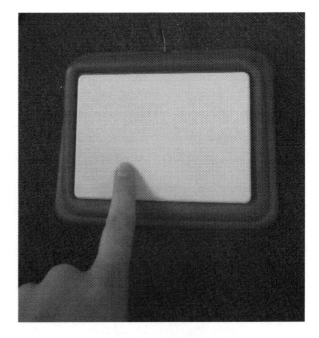

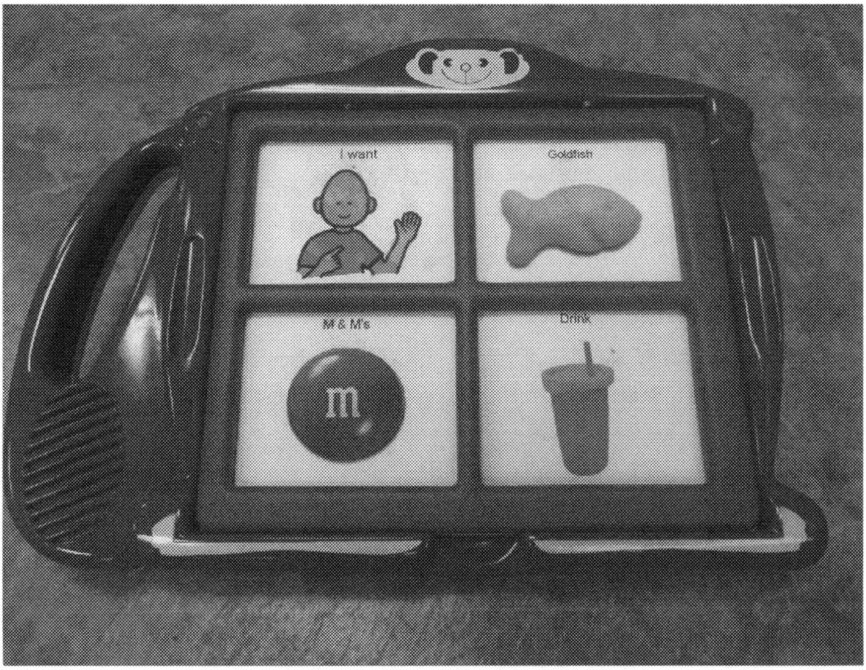

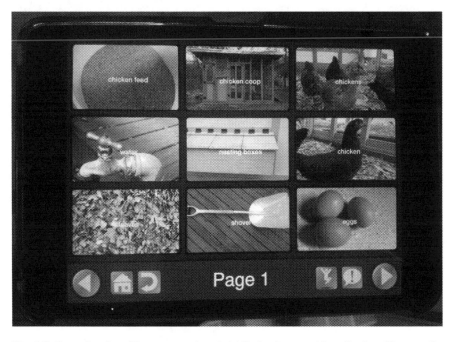

Fig. 2.4 Example of a four-choice array speech-generating device. Photo credit: Jennifer Ninci. Used with permission. The picture communication symbols ©1981–2010 by Mayer-Johnson LLC. All Rights Reserved Worldwide. Used with permission. Boardmaker™ is a trademark of Mayer-Johnson LLC

Fig. 2.5 Example of a tablet computer-based AAC nine-image grid application. Photo credit: Jennifer B. Ganz. Used with permission

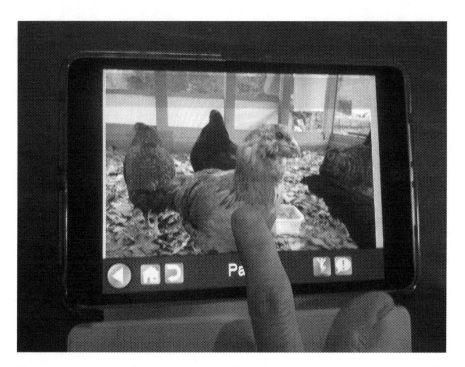

Fig. 2.6 Example of a visual scene display AAC page; the *shaded boxes* represent hot spots. Photo credit: Jennifer B. Ganz. Used with permission

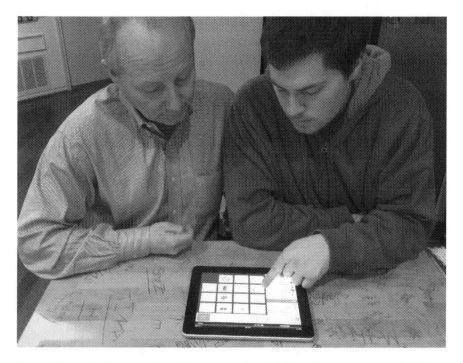

Fig. 2.7 Example of a man using a tablet computer-based AAC application. Photo credit: Margot B. Boles. Used with permission

disabilities that have CCN, are typically ambulatory (Sennott and Bowker 2009). Digital technologies are becoming more powerful while at the same time decreasing in size. Now, mobile devices are lightweight and can be used during various activities, including while seated at a table, but also while walking, riding in a car, or playing (Sennott and Bowker 2009). Further, dynamic mobile devices that make sound may be more appealing to many individuals with ASD than flat picture exchange systems (Ganz et al. 2013), leading to less abandonment of the system. Further, the speech output provides a consistent verbal model than low-tech AAC, increasing the opportunities for people with ASD to associate the spoken work with concrete concepts. Mobile device-based AAC also enables the person with CCN and others to quickly add vocabulary, which is not as easy when low-tech pictures must be located and printed (Ganz et al. 2013). Finally, because mobile devices are so ubiquitous, they may be more appealing than bulky communication books, which family members and teachers may feel are more noticeably "different." Indeed, teachers have reported that they preferred tablet computer-based AAC over picture exchange AAC, stating that they found it easier to use, took less preparation time, required fewer materials, and allowed students with ASD to communicate more quickly (Flores et al. 2012). Again, increasing the social validity and desirability of AAC may lead to more rapid adoption and lengthier use.

Types and Organization of Symbols Used in Aided AAC

AAC displays must take into account the age, functioning, and preferences of the person with ASD and CCN and his or her communicative partners (Light et al. 2007; Light and Drager 2002). Dynamic displays for AAC for mobile devices are available via computerized AAC programs and applications (for example, Dynavox Compass™,[1] Proloquo2Go[2]). That is, unlike traditional displays that had arrays that were fixed or that had to be manually moved, computerized apps and programs allow the user to organize and add vocabulary, incorporate new symbols and photos, automatically correct grammar and spelling, and have touch-screen capabilities, including swiping the screen to access additional vocabulary (Drager et al. 2004; Sennott and Bowker 2009). Traditionally, icons were displayed in grid arrays (Wilkinson and McIlvane 2013); however, now, they may also be provided in a format that incorporates contextual scene, called visual scene displays (VSDs), particularly thought to be useful for people with intellectual disabilities and young children with ASD.

VSDs are being promoted as a means of presenting concepts in a manner that more closely matches principles of visual processing to better enable people with CCN to communicate (Wilkinson and Jagaroo 2004). Unlike grid-style AAC

---

[1] www.mydynavox.com

[2] www.assistiveware.com

displays, VSDs have language concepts imbedded within photos or drawing of natural events (Wilkinson and Light 2011). These scenes are programmed with hot spots, so that components of the scenes say words or make sounds when tapped or selected (Wilkinson and Light 2011). For example, a photo of a child's house with the car parked in front may have hot spots that say, "window," when the window is touched and may make a sound of an engine revving when the image of the car is selected (Fig. 2.6 is an example of a VSD). Such an approach to presenting language appears to more closely match typical early language learning experiences, during which language is embedded in contextual experiences, rather than in isolation (Drager et al. 2003; Light et al. 2004). That is, typically developing children learn new vocabulary by hearing words in various contexts.

Several elements of VSDs are thought to be critical to providing access to AAC. One is attention to human figures (Wilkinson and Light 2011). Human figures have been found to draw visual attention in studies of typically developing individuals, regardless of the presence of other prominent objects (Wilkinson and Light 2011; Light and McNaughton 2012). Thus, it may be beneficial to include drawings or photos that have people in them. However, this may or may not be effective with individuals with ASD, given their decreased attention to humans when compared to attention to other objects in view (Klin et al. 2002; Riby and Hancock 2009). It should be noted though that individuals with ASD, while looking less at humans than their peers do, do look at humans at least some of the time (Riby and Hancock 2009), justifying the inclusion of human figures in at least some AAC displays. Two, vocabulary presented visually and in context appears to be easier to learn and identify than vocabulary presented in isolation in a grid format, particularly for very young children (Drager et al. 2003; Light and McNaughton 2012). That is, young children and older individuals with intellectual disabilities or significant language delays may benefit from the presentation of vocabulary in context and may learn to identify and locate that vocabulary on an AAC device more easily than in grid formats. Three, vocabulary is presented in a context that is familiar to the child (Light and McNaughton 2012); thus, children draw from memory of particular events to draw language concepts. Vocabulary in VSDs is presented similarly to the way in which children are exposed to new contexts in real life, through highly visual and complex contexts.

Although research has not yet been published that supports the use of VSDs with children with CCN, research has found that typically developing infants, finding they oriented to VSDs more than grid-type displays (Wilkinson and Light 2011) and that typically developing toddlers can locate concepts more easily on VSDs than grids (Drager et al. 2003).

Research Support for Aided AAC

Recent legislation requires that schools, and particularly special education programs, implement evidence-based practices (Reichow et al. 2008; Schlosser and Raghavendra 2004). In particular, meta-analytic procedures allow researchers to use a single metric to compare performance between baseline and intervention and to aggregate the results of numerous studies (Parker et al. 2009). A number of recent meta-analyses and literature reviews have been published summarizing the research on the use of aided AAC. Some of this work has focused exclusively or primarily on people with ASD, while other work has included a broader range of disability categories. This body of work provides some insight into the state of the field related to the effects of AAC.

AAC and ASD. Overall, via meta-analyses, AAC has been determined to be very effective in teaching communication skills to people with ASD (Ganz et al. 2012b). Further, meta-analyses have made more fine-grained analyses regarding the use of various types of AAC with people with ASD. More specifically, regarding particular outcomes, impacts on communication skills have been found to be greater than those for challenging behaviors and social interaction skills (Ganz et al. 2012b). When comparing effects on specific categories of outcomes related to what AAC mode was implemented, researchers found that communication outcomes were effected more by PECS and SGDs than other picture-based systems and that challenging behavior appeared to respond better to SGD interventions than PECS (Ganz et al. in press-b). These results should be interpreted with caution because of the small number of studies in each subcategory (e.g., effects of SGDs on challenging behaviors versus effects of PECS on challenging behaviors) and other factors that have not yet been investigated may be responsible. Comparisons across AAC mode have found that SGDs and PECS had significantly better overall effects than other types of picture-based AAC (Ganz et al. 2012b). Participant characteristics also had some impact on the efficacy of aided AAC interventions (Ganz et al. 2011a). Specifically, individuals with ASD and no comorbid disabilities had better outcomes than those with ASD and ID, and young children had better outcomes than older individuals with ASD. Further, AAC was more effective in general education settings than others (Ganz et al. in press-b), potentially related to the functioning level of the individuals with ASD who are more likely to be placed in general education settings; however, this is unclear in the current research literature.

Additionally, meta-analyses and literature reviews have focused on individual AAC modes, including PECS and SGDs, used with people with ASD. Ganz et al. (2012a) conducted a meta-analysis on the impact of PECS on outcomes in individuals with ASD, finding that PECS had moderate overall effects. Further, effects were moderate for targeted AAC-use outcome measures (i.e., learning to use pictures to request) and weaker for non-targeted skills (i.e., collateral outcomes that are not specifically aims of PECS), such as challenging behavior, social interactions, and speech. Further, PECS was more effective on targeted outcomes for preschool children than elementary-aged children; the number of studies with older individuals was too small to make a confident comparison. Additional meta-analyses and literature reviews on the use of PECS and SGDs with people with ASD have been published (Flippin et al. 2010; Ostryn et al. 2008; Preston and Carter 2009; van der Meer and Rispoli 2010); due to their use of discredited metrics for meta-analysis, such as PND (Subramanian and Wendt 2010), or no effect size measures, their results must be interpreted with caution. However, when considered as a whole, they provide support for the statement that the majority of participants who were taught PECS and SGDs had gains in AAC use.

AAC and DD. Only one recent meta-analysis has been conducted using up-to-date effect size metrics to investigate the impact of AAC on people with DD overall; though there have been additional reviews that have also considered this topic. Walker and Snell (2013) conducted a meta-analysis of the impact of all types of AAC on challenging behaviors. Findings indicated that overall, AAC interventions result in decreased challenging behaviors in individuals with CCN. In particular, interventions incorporating functional behavior assessment had stronger effects on challenging behavior than those that did not. Further, AAC was more effective on challenging behaviors in younger children than older individuals, although far fewer studies were conducted with adults than children. Other reviews have been conducted, but should be considered with caution because their chosen metric, percent of non-overlapping data (PND; Scruggs et al. 1986), is limited in that PND values cannot be aggregated into overall effect sizes (Subramanian and Wendt 2010) or because they only provide summaries of the literature without an aggregating metric that meets current standards.

When investigating the impact of AAC on outcome measures (i.e., targeted skills) in people with DD, findings of less rigorous reviews have been positive for communication and other outcomes. Lancioni et al. (2007) reviewed the literature on the use of picture exchange systems and SGDs to teach requesting to people with DD, finding that most participants were successfully taught to communicate, regardless of the selected AAC mode, and participants did not significantly select one over the other when given the choice. Although families often express concern that AAC will inhibit speech, reviews have suggested that none of the studies reported decreased speech and most found speech gains occurred as AAC was implemented (Ganz et al. 2008b, 2010a, 2011b; Hart and Banda 2010; Millar et al. 2006). Further, Chung and colleagues' (2012) review suggested that overall, the effects were positive for peer interaction during AAC interventions.

Reviews that investigated or compared particular AAC modes have concluded that they are effective with people with DD. SGDs have been successfully implemented with people with DD (Rispoli et al. 2010). A review of PECS implementation suggested that PECS had positive outcomes related to communication, particularly the use of AAC for requesting, and some participants had improvements in social interaction and challenging behaviors (Sulzer-Azaroff et al. 2009). However, this article included studies that did not meet minimum quality criteria and should be interpreted with caution because most studies included only evaluated half or fewer of the PECS instructional phases. Further, four of the five authors were employees of Pyramid Educational Consultants, who sell PECS materials and provide training, including the two developers of PECS; thus, the authors had a conflict of interest. Therefore, the results of this review should be interpreted with caution, although their results are reflective of those found in more rigorous meta-analyses (Ganz, et al. 2012a).

A few reviews have reviewed literature relevant to participant choice of AAC system. Investigations of preference of people with CCN have indicated that they tend to prefer aided AAC to unaided; however, this may relate to the level of motor imitation skills in the individual or other individual characteristics (Gevarter et al. 2013). Further, van der Meer et al. (2011) evaluated studies that assessed preference across mode of AAC, including manual sign, picture exchange-based systems, and SGDs, finding that more of the participant preferred SGDs, although many others preferred picture exchange.

Conclusions and Future Research Directions

It is clear that aided AAC has a history of effective implementation with people with ASD, particularly in teaching requesting skills, and for young children with ASD (Ganz et al. 2012b). Aided AAC is a potential alternative for individuals who cannot communicate effectively with speech (Romski and Sevcik 1997). However, there remain numerous questions regarding for whom AAC is most effective and matching AAC to client characteristics, new modes and formats of AAC, comparisons across modes of AAC and related to client preference, key implementation strategies, and generalization and maintenance of learned skills across natural contexts.

Research has primarily involved a limited range of participant characteristics. Across meta-analyses and literature reviews, authors noted that the majority of research on AAC, including those with participants with ASD, have involved children (Chung et al. 2012; Ganz et al. 2012b). Thus, it is critical that more research with young adults and adults with CCN be conducted. In particular, it is critical to determine if particular strategies may be implemented with older individuals to raise the effectiveness of AAC to levels seen in preschool children (Ganz et al. 2011a) and to determine if strategies or AAC modes need to be adapted to be more effective for individuals with comorbid disabilities, such as sensory impairments. Research on the use of aided AAC with individuals from culturally and linguistically diverse backgrounds is lacking (Ganz et al. 2012c; Simpson and Ganz 2012). As the USA becomes more diverse, it becomes more imperative to investigate the impact of various languages of instruction on individuals who come from homes in which the primary language is different from that of the school they attend or community in which they live. Finally, instructional modifications for individuals who do not learn to use AAC as rapidly as most should be investigated (Ganz et al. 2005; Ganz et al. 2010b).

The variety and availability of modes of AAC are rapidly expanding to include lower-priced applications for mobile technology. Because the use of these devices is relatively new, few published studies have incorporated them. Investigations involving complex AAC systems, such as those with dynamic displays, are needed (Chung et al. 2012; Drager et al. 2004; Ganz et al. in press-a). In particular, research that investigates the feasibility of use of high-tech AAC for caregivers, practitioners, and people with CCN is lacking. Research investigating new AAC applications that are flexible in the creation of new vocabulary in the moment and that are usable for all stakeholders would be helpful. Currently, low-tech aided AAC may be preferable due to its cost-effectiveness, portability, and ease of repair compared to higher-tech devices (Wilkinson and Hennig 2007); however, as prices for portable electronics drop, this may change.

Articles that have investigated comparisons between AAC modes and related to personal preference for particular AAC mode are increasing in the literature; however, such work is still needed. Gevarter et al. (2013) concluded that comparative research, including aided AAC, unaided AAC, and speech-based instruction, is still needed. Further, the role of preference of AAC mode by the person with CCN should be investigated further (Ganz et al. 2013; Sigafoos et al. 2005; van der Meer et al. 2011), particularly in terms of impact on outcomes and how to best evaluate preference when selecting a device or mode.

Finally, future research is needed to investigate expanding treatment techniques and broad demonstration of skills across varied natural contexts. Much of the literature is limited to primary communication outcomes and highly structured settings. Intervention strategies cited in research vary widely, from highly structured protocols to sparsely described procedures; research should be conducted to answer questions related to the best combination of strategies to meet the needs of people with CCN. While the type of AAC used is important, more important is discovering specific strategies that can be used across AAC types to improve outcomes of people with ASD and CCN. Further, because much of the research involves implementation by highly trained researchers, research involving implementation of AAC strategies by typical service providers and caregivers (Chung et al. 2012) under typical circumstances is needed, including investigations of feasibility of implementation and treatment fidelity (Hart and Banda 2010), or how well typical communicative partners can implement interventions. Further, studies are needed that investigate more advanced AAC skills, as most studies on people with ASD have evaluated impacts only on requesting (Ganz et al. 2012a). This research base would benefit from measures of the effects of AAC generalized across contexts and maintained long term (Didden 2012; Ganz et al. 2008a; Hart and Banda 2010), which is unfortunately missing from much of the single-case research on AAC to date.

References

Bondy, A. (2012). The unusual suspects: Myths and misconceptions associated with PECS. *Psychological Record, 62*, 789–816.

Bondy, A., & Frost, L. (1994). The Picture Exchange Communication System. *Focus on Autistic Behavior, 9*, 1–19.

Chung, Y., Carter, E. W., & Sisco, L. G. (2012). A systematic review of interventions to increase peer interactions for students with complex communication challenges. *Research and Practice for Persons with Severe Disabilities, 37*, 271–287.

Didden, R. (2012). Participant and intervention characteristics influence the effectiveness of the picture exchange communication system (PECS) for children with ASD1. *Evidence-Based Communication Assessment and Intervention, 6*, 174–176. doi:10.1080/17489539.2013.771885.

Drager, K. D. R., Light, J. C., Carlson, R., D'Silva, K., Larsson, B., Pitkin, L., & Stopper, G. (2004). Learning of dynamic display AAC technologies by typically developing 3-year-olds: Effect of different layouts and menu approaches. *Journal of Speech, Language, and Hearing Research, 47*, 1133–1148. doi:10.1044/1092-4388(2004/084)

Drager, K. D. R., Light, J. C., Speltz, J. C., Fallon, K. A., & Jeffries, L. Z. (2003). The performance of typically developing 2 1/2-year-olds on dynamic display AAC technologies with different system layouts and language organizations. *Journal of Speech, Language, and Hearing Research, 46,* 298–312.

Flippin, M., Reszka, S., & Watson, L. R. (2010). Effectiveness of the picture exchange communication system (PECS) on communication and speech for children with autism spectrum disorders: A meta-analysis. *American Journal of Speech-Language Pathology, 19,* 178–195. doi:10.1044/1058-0360(2010/09-0022).

Flores, M., Musgrove, K., Renner, S., Hinton, V., Strozier, S., Franklin, S., & Hil, D. (2012). A comparison of communication using the Apple iPad and a picture-based system. *Augmentative and Alternative Communication, 28,* 74–84. doi:10.3109/07434618.2011.644579

Frost, L., & Bondy, A. (2002). *The Picture Exchange Communication System (PECS) training manual* (2nd ed.). Newark, NJ: DE: Pyramid Publications.

Gal, E., Bauminger, N., Goren-Bar, D., Pianesi, F., Stock, O., Zancanaro, M., & Weiss, P. L. T. (2009). Enhancing social communication of children with high-functioning autism through a co-located interface. *AI & Society, 24,* 75–84. doi: 10.1007/s00146-009-0199-0.

Ganz, J. B., Boles, M. B., Goodwyn, F. D., & Flores, M. M. (2014). Efficacy of handheld electronic visual supports to enhance vocabulary in children with ASD. *Focus on Autism and Other Developmental Disabilities, 29,* 3–12. doi: 10.1177/108835761350491.

Ganz, J. B., Cook, K. E., Corbin-Newsome, J., Bourgeois, B., & Flores, M. (2005). Variations on the use of a pictorial alternative communication system with a child with autism and developmental delays. *TEACHING Exceptional Children Plus, 1,* Article 3. Retrieved from http://escholarship.bc.edu/education/tecplus/vol1/iss6/art3/

Ganz, J. B., Davis, J. L., Lund, E. M., Goodwyn, F. D., & Simpson, R. L. (2012a). Meta-analysis of PECS with individuals with ASD: Investigation of targeted versus non-targeted outcomes, participant characteristics, and implementation phase. *Research in Developmental Disabilities, 33,* 406–418. doi: 10.1016/j.ridd.2011.09.023

Ganz, J. B., Earles-Vollrath, T. L., Heath, A. K., Parker, R. I., Rispoli, M. J., & Duran, J. B. (2012b). A meta-analysis of single case research studies on aided augmentative and alternative communication systems with individuals with autism spectrum disorders. *Journal of Autism and Developmental Disorders, 42,* 60–74. doi: 10.1007/s10803-011-1212-2

Ganz, J. B., Earles-Vollrath, T. L., Mason, R. A., Rispoli, M. J., Heath, A. K., & Parker, R. I. (2011a). An aggregate study of single-case research involving aided AAC: Participant characteristics of individuals with autism spectrum disorders. *Research in Autism Spectrum Disorders, 5,* 1500–1509. doi: 10.1016/j.rasd.2011.02.011

Ganz, J. B., Flores, M. M., & Lashley, E. (2011b). Effects of a treatment package on imitated and spontaneous verbal requests in children with autism. *Education and Training in Autism and Developmental Disabilities, 46,* 596–606.

Ganz, J. B., Heath, A. K., Rispoli, M. J., & Earles-Vollrath, T. (2010a). Impact of AAC versus verbal modeling on verbal imitation, picture discrimination, and related speech: A pilot investigation. *Journal of Developmental and Physical Disabilities, 22,* 179–196. doi:10.1007/s10882-009-9176-2.

Ganz, J. B., Hong, E. R., & Goodwyn, F. D. (2013). Effectiveness of the PECS phase III app and choice between the app and traditional PECS among preschoolers with ASD. *Research in Autism Spectrum Disorders, 7,* 973–983. doi:10.1016/j.rasd.2013.04.003.

Ganz, J. B., Hong, E. R, Goodwyn, F. D., Kite, E., & Gilliland, W. (in press-a). Impact of PECS tablet computer app on receptive identification of pictures given a verbal stimulus. *Developmental Neurorehabilitation.* doi: 10.3109/17518423.2013.821539

Ganz, J. B., Lashley, E., & Rispoli, M. J. (2010b). Non-responsiveness to intervention: Children with autism spectrum disorders who do not rapidly respond to communication interventions. *Developmental Neurorehabilitation, 13,* 399–407.

Ganz, J. B., Rispoli, M. J., Mason, R. A., & Hong, E. R. (in press-b). Moderation of effects of AAC based on setting and types of aided AAC on outcome variables: An aggregate study of single-case research with individuals with ASD. *Developmental Neurorehabilitation.* doi: 10.3109/17518423.2012.748097

Ganz, J. B., Sigafoos, J., Simpson, R. L., & Cook, K.E. (2008a). Generalization of a pictorial alternative communication system across instructors and distance. *Augmentative and Alternative Communication, 24*, 89–99.

Ganz, J. B., Simpson, R. L., & Corbin-Newsome, J. (2008b). The impact of the Picture Exchange Communication System on requesting and speech development in preschoolers with autism spectrum disorders and similar characteristics. *Research in Autism Spectrum Disorders, 2*, 157–169. doi: 10.1016/j.rasd.2007.04.005

Ganz, J. B., Simpson, R. L., & Lund, E. M. (2012c). The picture exchange communication system (PECS): A promising method for improving communication skills of learners with autism spectrum disorders. *Education and Training in Autism and Developmental Disabilities, 47*, 176–186.

Gevarter, C., O'Reilly, M. F., Rojeski, L., Sammarco, N., Lang, R., Lancioni, G. E., & Sigafoos, J. (2013). Comparisons of intervention components within augmentative and alternative communication systems for individuals with developmental disabilities: A review of the literature. *Research in Developmental Disabilities, 34*(12), 4404–4414. doi:10.1016/j.ridd.2013.09.018

Hart, S. L., & Banda, D. R. (2010). Picture exchange communication system with individuals with developmental disabilities: A meta-analysis of single subject studies. *Remedial and Special Education, 31*, 476–488. doi:10.1177/0741932509338354.

Kagohara, D. M., van der Meer, L., Ramdoss, S., O'Reilly, M. F., Lancioni, G. E., Davis, T. N., … Sigafoos, J. (2013). Using iPods® and iPads® in teaching programs for individuals with developmental disabilities: A systematic review. *Research in Developmental Disabilities, 34*, 147–156. doi:10.1016/j.ridd.2012.07.027

Klin, A., Jones, W., Schultz, R., Volkmar, F., & Cohen, D. (2002). Visual fixation patterns during viewing of naturalistic social situation as predictors of social competence in individuals with autism. *Archives of General Psychiatry, 59*, 809–816.

Lancioni, G. E., O'Reilly, M. F., Cuvo, A. J., Singh, N. N., Sigafoos, J., & Didden, R. (2007). PECS and VOCAs to enable students with developmental disabilities to make requests: An overview of the literature. *Research in Developmental Disabilities, 28*, 468–488. doi:10.1016/j.ridd.2006.06.003.

Light, J. C., & Drager, K. D. (2002). Improving the design of augmentative and alternative technologies for young children. *Assistive Technology, 14*, 17–32.

Light, J., Drager, K., McCarthy, J., Mellott, S., Millar, D., Parrish, C., … Welliver, M. (2004). Performance of typically developing four- and five-year-old children with AAC systems using different language organization techniques. *Augmentative and Alternative Communication, 20*, 63–88.

Light, J., & McNaughton, D. (2012). Supporting the communication, language, and literacy development of children with complex communication needs: State of the science and future research priorities. *Assistive Technology, 24*, 34–44.

Light, J., Page, R., Curran, J., & Pitkin, L. (2007). Children's ideas for the design of AAC assistive technologies for young children with complex communication needs. *Augmentative and Alternative Communication, 23*, 274–287. doi:10.1080/07434610701390475.

Light, J. C., Roberts, B., Dimarco, R., & Greiner, N. (1998). Augmentative and alternative communication to support receptive and expressive communication for people with autism. *Journal of Communication Disorders, 31*, 153–180.

McNaughton, D., & Light, J. (2013). The iPad and mobile technology revolution: Benefits and challenges for individuals who require augmentative and alternative communication. *Augmentative and Alternative Communication, 29*, 107–116. doi:10.3109/07434618.2013.784930.

Millar, D. C., Light, J. C., & Schlosser, R. W. (2006). The impact of augmentative and alternative communication intervention on the speech production of individuals with developmental disabilities: A research review. *Journal of Speech, Language, and Hearing Research, 49*, 248–264. doi:10.1044/1092-4388(2006/021).

Murdock, L. C., Ganz, J. B., & Crittenden, J. (2013). Use of an iPad play story to increase play dialog of preschoolers with autism spectrum disorders. *Journal of Autism and Developmental Disorders, 43*, 2174–2189. doi:10.1007/s10803-013-1770-6.

Ostryn, C., Wolfe, P. S., & Rusch, F. R. (2008). A review and analysis of the picture exchange communication system (PECS) for individuals with autism spectrum disorders using a paradigm of communication competence. *Research and Practice for Persons with Severe Disabilities, 33*, 13–24.

Parker, R. I., Vannest, K. J., & Brown, L. (2009). The improvement rate difference for single case research. *Exceptional Children, 75*, 135–150.

Preston, D., & Carter, M. (2009). A review of the efficacy of the picture exchange communication system intervention. *Journal of Autism and Developmental Disorders, 39*, 1471–1486. doi:10.1007/s10803-009-0763-y.

Reichow, B., Volkmar, F. R., & Cicchetti, D. V. (2008). Development of the evaluative methods for evaluating and determining evidence-based practices in autism. *Journal of Autism and Developmental Disorders, 28*, 1311–1319.

Riby, D., & Hancock, P. J. B. (2009). Do faces capture the attention of individuals with Williams syndrome or autism? *Neuropsychologia, 46*, 2855–2860.

Rispoli, M. J., Franco, J. H., van der Meer, L., Lang, R., & Camargo, S. P. (2010). The use of speech generating devices in communication interventions for individuals with developmental disabilities: A review of the literature. *Developmental Neurorehabilitation, 13*, 276–293.

Romski, M. A., & Sevcik, R. A. (1997). Augmentative and alternative communication for children with developmental disabilities. *Mental Retardation and Developmental Disabilities Research Reviews, 3*, 363–368.

Schepis, M. M., Reid, D. H., Behrmann, M. M., & Sutton, K. A. (1998). Increasing communicative interactions of young children with autism using a voice output communication aid and naturalistic teaching. *Journal of Applied Behavior Analysis, 31*, 561–578. doi:10.1901/jaba.1998.31-561.

Schlosser, R. W., & Raghavendra, P. (2004). Evidence-based practice in augmentative and alternative communication. *Augmentative and Alternative Communication, 20*, 1–21. doi:10.1080/07434610310001621083.

Scruggs, T., Mastropieri, M., Cook, S., & Escobar, C. (1986). Early intervention for children with conduct disorders: A quantitative synthesis of single-subject research. *Behavioral Disorders, 11*, 260–271.

Sennott, S., & Bowker, A. (2009). Autism, AAC, and Proloquo2Go. *Perspectives on Augmentative and Alternative Communication, 18*, 137–145. doi:10.1044/aac18.4.137.

Shane, H. C., Laubscher, E. H., Schlosser, R. W., Flynn, S., Sorce, J. F., & Abramson, J. (2012). Applying technology to visually support language and communication in individuals with autism spectrum disorders. *Journal of Autism and Developmental Disorders, 42*, 1228–1235. doi:10.1007/s10803-011-1304-z.

Sigafoos, J., O'Reilly, M., Ganz, J. B., Lancioni, G. E., & Schlosser, R. W. (2005). Supporting self-determination in AAC interventions by assessing preferences for communication devices. *Technology and Disability, 17*, 143–153.

Simpson, R. L., & Ganz, J. B. (2012). The Picture Exchange Communication System (PECS). In P. Prelock & R. McCauley (Eds.), *Treatment of autism spectrum disorders: Evidence-based intervention strategies for communication & social interaction* (pp. 255–280). Baltimore: Paul H Brookes Publishing.

Skinner, B. F. (1957). *Verbal behavior*. Englewood Cliffs, NJ: Prentice Hall.

Son, S., Sigafoos, J., O'Reilly, M., & Lancioni, G. E. (2006). Comparing two types of augmentative and alternative communication systems for children with autism. *Pediatric Rehabilitation, 9*, 389–395. doi:10.1080/13638490500519984.

Subramanian, A., & Wendt, O. (2010). PECS has empirical support, but limitations in the systematic review process require this conclusion to be interpreted with caution. *Evidence-Based Communication Assessment and Intervention, 4*, 22–26. doi:10.1080/17489530903550341.

Sulzer-Azaroff, B., Hoffman, A. O., Horton, C. B., Bondy, A., & Frost, L. (2009). The picture exchange communication system (PECS): What do the data say? *Focus on Autism and Other Developmental Disabilities, 24*, 89–103. doi:10.1177/1088357609332743.

van der Meer, L. A. J., & Rispoli, M. (2010). Communication interventions involving speech-generating devices for children with autism: A review of the literature. *Developmental Neurorehabilitation, 13*, 294–306. doi:2048/10.3109/17518421003671494.

van der Meer, L., Sigafoos, J., O'Reilly, M. F., & Lancioni, G. E. (2011). Assessing preferences for AAC options in communication interventions for individuals with developmental disabilities: A review of the literature. *Research in Developmental Disabilities, 32*, 1422–1431. doi:10.1016/j.ridd.2011.02.003.

van der Meer, L., Sutherland, D., O'Reilly, M. F., Lancioni, G. E., & Sigafoos, J. (2012). A further comparison of manual signing, picture exchange, and speech-generating devices as communication modes for children with autism spectrum disorders. *Research in Autism Spectrum Disorders, 6*, 1247–1257.

Walker, V. L., & Snell, M. E. (2013). Effects of augmentative and alternative communication on challenging behavior: A meta-analysis. *Augmentative and Alternative Communication, 29*, 117–131. doi:10.3109/07434618.2013.785020.

Wilkinson, K. M., & Hennig, S. (2007). The state of research and practice in augmentative and alternative communication for children with developmental/intellectual disabilities. *Mental Retardation and Developmental Disabilities Research Reviews, 13*, 58–69. doi:10.1002/nrdd.2013.

Wilkinson, K. M., & Jagaroo, V. (2004). Contributions of principles of visual cognitive science to AAC system display design. *Augmentative and Alternative Communication, 20*, 123–136.

Wilkinson, K. M., & Light, J. (2011). Preliminary investigation of visual attention to human figures in photographs: Potential considerations for the design of aided AAC visual scene displays. *Journal of Speech, Language, and Hearing Research, 54*, 1644–1657. doi:10.1044/1092-4388(2011/10-0098).

Wilkinson, K. M., & McIlvane, W. J. (2013). Perceptual factors influence visual search for meaningful symbols in individuals with intellectual disabilities and Down syndrome or autism spectrum disorders. *American Journal on Intellectual and Developmental Disabilities, 118*, 353–364. doi:10.1352/1944-7558-118.5.353.

Chapter 3
AAC and Assessment of People with ASD and CCN

Parents and other stakeholders often question whether aided augmentative and alternative communication (AAC) is appropriate for their loved one who has autism spectrum disorder (ASD) and complex communication need (CCN). In particular, aided AAC is suitable for individuals who do not currently have an effective functional communication method or have difficulty being understood by others via speech (Pyramid Educational Consultants 2013). Those with difficulty communicating verbally and who have challenging behavior may be particularly well suited for AAC, which may diminish the need for problematic behavior by providing an effective means to communicate (Ganz et al. 2009). People who have difficulty with joint attention (e.g., sharing interests in objects or ideas with others), who have strong interests in objects, and who have poor motor skills may be suitable for aided AAC (Flippin et al. 2010; Ganz et al. 2012; Simpson and Ganz 2012). Further, because aided AAC systems are inherently visual in nature, they may be particularly suited to people with ASD many of whom have strengths in interpreting information provided visually, reducing abstract thinking requirements inherent in less iconic language systems, such as verbal and sign language systems (Ganz et al. 2012; Heflin and Alaimo 2007; Mirenda 2001).

Evaluation is necessary to determine whether or not to implement aided AAC and to determine goals; however, assessment of individuals who do not communicate in traditional manners is complicated by the fact that many direct assessment tools require examinees to provide verbal responses (Lund et al. in press). Questions regarding the selection of an alternative communication modality challenge both families and professionals. Thus, this chapter provides practical information regarding assessments and procedures aimed at selecting an aided AAC system/mode for people with ASD and CCNs and methods of evaluating the skills of individuals with ASD and CCN. The evaluations discussed in this chapter relate only to assessments and related issues for evaluating skill levels and for the purpose of selecting AAC; this chapter does not address diagnostic assessments nor is it a manual for standard assessment practices. The information herein is intended to provide an overview of AAC assessment concepts and practical information for

J.B. Ganz, *Aided Augmentative Communication for Individuals with Autism Spectrum Disorders*, Autism and Child Psychopathology Series, DOI 10.1007/978-1-4939-0814-1_3,
© Springer Science+Business Media New York 2014

professionals, practitioners, and families. All assessments should be conducted by an individual who is qualified to do so, as specified in most assessment manuals. That is, this chapter is intended to provide guidance, particularly toward determining the appropriateness of and selecting aided AAC. Specific assessments are described as examples; specific assessments for a given individual should be carefully selected by his or her interdisciplinary team, including those with particular expertise in psychology and communication disorders.

AAC assessment requires a team of professionals with varied areas of expertise (Batorowicz and Shepherd 2011; Dietz et al. 2012). AAC assessment teams typically include speech-language pathologists, educators, family members, the person with ASD when appropriate, and, if there are medical needs, medical professionals (Dietz et al. 2012). At least one member of the team should be aware and knowledgeable about current and rapidly increasing technological options in AAC and should have experience and training related to implementation of AAC (Dietz et al. 2012). More details regarding collaboration among professionals in varied disciplines are discussed in Chap. 4.

Evaluating to Select an Aided AAC System

Assessments to determine the suitability of AAC and to select a system and relevant goals should include formal tools, informal tools and observations, and professional judgment (Flippin et al. 2010; Ganz et al. 2012; Ogletree 2008; Simpson and Ganz 2012). Prior to formal assessment, AAC assessment teams should conduct a case history to gather information related to the client/student's educational, family, and social history, as well as what the individual's communication needs and motivations are (Dietz et al. 2012). Information should be gathered on the individual's motor, cognitive, literacy, and communication skills to enable the evaluators to prepare materials and devices that might be tried and gather appropriate assessment tools. The following are common approaches and components of AAC assessment. Specific communication assessments are discussed later in this chapter.

Social and Communication Assessment. Social and communication assessments should be conducted that include investigations of the individual's receptive language (i.e., language comprehension), expressive language (i.e., language output), oral-motor, reading, writing skills, and social interactions and needs (Calculator and Black 2009; Dietz et al. 2012); recommendations regarding specific language and communication assessments are given below. Evaluations should include direct observation in and information about use of language in natural contexts. That is, a full range of a person's need to communicate across contexts should be considered, such as in personal interactions, in school assignments and educational settings, and via technology and the Internet (Light and McNaughton 2012).

In particular, Light (1997) recommends that physical, functional, language, social, and cultural contexts of the individual's language learning environment be evaluated and later addressed in intervention. Assessment of the *physical context* of language learning involves defining and describing the items, people, and events in the person's environment (Light 1997).

Evaluating the *functional context* includes determining the time, place, structure, and function of interactions within the person's daily activities (Light 1997). In particular, assessment of functional context includes describing when language is facilitated throughout the day, when language intervention would not be ideal due to other demands, when the individual is free from structured activities, and when additional language instructions could occur (von Tetzchner and Martinsen 1992). By defining activities throughout the individual's day during which language may be used provide opportunities to discover when use of AAC may be expanded or used to address communicative breakdowns.

Assessment of the *language context* includes examining the communication modes and symbols in use by the individual with CCN, his or her family, and others with whom he or she interacts regularly (Light 1997). In addition to the formal assessments described below, evaluating the language context of the individual should include informal observations of natural contexts. This should include the person's understanding of language in the person's current and likely future daily environments and activities to determine the necessity of augmenting his or her input, or whether or not augmentative means may be necessary to improve his or her understanding of the communication used by others. Further, the person's expressive communication should be evaluated in natural contexts to determine the various forms of communication the person already uses; that is, as discussed below, a combination of modes, such as speech approximations, AAC symbols, and gestures, may be an appropriate approach, building on the person's current skills as determined by formal and informal assessments (Light 1997). Further, assessment of the language context should include a description of the person's current and needed vocabulary and syntactic skills.

Evaluation of the *social context* includes investigations of interactions between the person with CCN and others, including communication barriers that exist (Light 1997). Social functioning and friendship should be evaluated, with an eye toward determining skills necessary to promote making and maintaining friendships (Calculator and Black 2009). Further, informal assessment may determine how others in the environment may scaffold communication skills and how this support may be faded to provide the individual with more opportunities to independently and spontaneously communicate and direct communicative interactions (Light 1997). Turn-taking and modeling of language may occur or the assessment may uncover additional opportunities to model use of communication, including AAC-based communication, which will be discussed further in Chap. 5.

Evaluating the *cultural context* involves describing values, beliefs, and expectations of the person's family, community, and other stakeholders (Light 1997). Assessment may include informal discussion with stakeholders regarding their priorities for the individual's communication development, preferred device(s), and multimodal use of communication skills.

Assessment of Symbol Comprehension and Use. AAC assessments should include evaluation of the individual's ability to use and comprehend communication and

symbolic language, particularly related to symbols that may be used in AAC devices
(Dietz et al. 2012). Young children, preliterate individuals, and those with more
significant intellectual disabilities may be best able to comprehend images with
high iconicity, or a strong relationship between the image and the item or concept
represented (e.g., photographs), and those symbols that represent concrete concepts
like nouns (Light and McNaughton 2012). Recent research suggests that animated
symbols may be particularly appealing and comprehensible to some individuals
with CCN (Jagaroo and Wilkinson 2008; Mineo et al. 2008). In addition to evaluating the types of symbols that may be appropriate for a given individual (e.g., written
words, line drawings), it is important to evaluate the type of display appropriate,
such as a grid format versus visual scene displays, appeal of the system to the family
of and person with ASD, and the efficiency and accessibility of categorical or the-
matic organization of vocabulary within the system (Dietz et al. 2012; Light and
McNaughton 2012). Unfortunately, little guidance exists related to the decision-
making process professionals use when selecting displayed appropriate for clients
(McFadd and Wilkinson 2010). Research related to symbolic representation and
organization is discussed in more detail in Chap. 2.

Selection of AAC. Another step is selection of one or more modes of AAC to try with
the individual with ASD and CCN. When selecting particular modes of AAC to
implement with an individual, several variables should be considered, particularly
when the individual has challenging behaviors that need to be addressed via functional communication training (see Chap. 7) (Heath 2012; Ringdahl et al. 2009). One,
the amount of effort necessary to produce the AAC behavior should be considered
(Ringdahl et al. 2009). That is, it may take significantly more effort for the person to
navigate through a multipage SGD app to compose a complex message while the
same message may be given with a single icon on a home page instead (Bailey et al.
2002). This may be particularly important if the new communication form is aimed
at replacing a severe behavior, which may have been reinforced for many years. For
example, if a child with ASD made a loud shriek when peers came close, resulting in
them moving away, it may be more appropriate to give him a single-switch SGD that
stated, "GIVE ME SPACE, PLEASE," with a single button than expecting him to
compose a message using several icons on a tablet computer-based AAC app.

Two, the novelty of the AAC behavior may increase the likelihood that the person will be willing to use that mode (Heath 2012; Ringdahl et al. 2009; Winborn-
Kemmerer et al. 2010). For example, newer technologies may be more appealing to
the person adopting a new AAC mode because they may be different from paper–
pencil tasks or desktop computer programs they are used to. Three, the intellectual
functioning of the individual may indicate that more or less complex AAC systems
might be appropriate (DeRuyter and Becker 1988). That is, an individual with more
severe intellectual disabilities along with ASD might benefit more from a system
that requires less system navigation, while someone with average or better intelligence may be able to navigate through multiple pages and levels to form messages.
Four, the individual's proficiency with the communicative mode should be considered (Heath 2012; Ringdahl et al. 2009). If the new communication behavior is

easily performed by the individual and results in quick access to reinforcement, he or she is more likely to continue engaging in that behavior.

Five, the preference of the individual and his or her family should be considered. Researchers have suggested that preference assessments be performed, by allowing the individual to choose which system to use (Sigafoos et al. 2009; van der Meer et al. 2011). The instructor may place a number of options in front of the person and allow him or her to take the device he or she would like to use. Such assessments may be performed after initial instruction is given in the use of each system and may be performed periodically to determine if preferences have changed (Cannella-Malone et al. 2009; Stafford et al. 2002). More information regarding the involvement of family members in decision-making is provided in Chap. 4.

Multimodal Communication. AAC evaluators emphasize the need for a multimodal approach to communication (DeRuyter and Becker 1988; Dietz et al. 2012; Light 1997). That is, individuals with CCN may need different options for different environments or contexts, including natural speech, speech approximations, AAC devices, gestures, and facial expressions (Light 1997). For example, nodding yes or no may be the most efficient means of answering some questions, low-tech concrete picture systems may be lightweight and appropriate for the community, while higher-tech devices may be needed for more complex communication in the classroom or home. Further, speech should be used in concert with AAC, whether through speech-generating devices or as modeled by practitioners and caregivers (Light 1997). More information on the combination of AAC with speech for receptive and expressive communication instruction is provided in Chap. 5.

AAC Device Trials and Operational Demands. Once one or more devices and symbol systems are tentatively selected, AAC assessments should include evaluation of the operational demands of potential AAC systems, including trials with a variety of devices to determine which device works best for that individual, is most efficient and effective, and if symbols are appropriate or need to be reorganized (Dietz et al. 2012; Light 1997). Further, assessments and trials may determine whether or not the person with CCN has ready access to AAC in all necessary contexts (Light 1997). Relatedly, assessments should include a means for determining the preferences of family members of and individuals with CCN for particular AAC modes (Calculator and Black 2009). Chapter 4 provides more insight into collaboration with family members and individuals with ASD and CCN to determine preferences and the impact of AAC on their daily lives.

Assessment of Students with ASD Who Use AAC

Tools for Selection of Specific AAC Modes

There are limited formal evaluation tools designed specifically for the purpose of assessing issues related to symbol selection for AAC. One is the Test of Aided-communication Symbol Performance (TASP; Bruno 2006). It evaluates four areas, including symbol size and quantity, grammar, categorization of symbols, and syntax. The symbols are presented in a grid format and using picture communication symbols (PCS), which is a widely used AAC picture set (Dynavox Mayer-Johnson 1981–2009; McDougall et al. 2012). Further, the TASP may be efficient because it takes only 10–20 min to administer (Bruno 2006). In one study, the TASP was successfully implemented in computerized format, although only one participant had ASD (McDougall et al. 2012). While it may provide some information relevant to AAC evaluations, the TASP has some limitations, including the reliance on grid formatting (versus inclusion of animated symbols and visual scene displays), the requirement that the examinee must be able to make selections via pointing, the use of a singular type of symbol (e.g., line drawings and photos only), individuals with ASD who have never used AAC before may not understand the task directions and may score at the basal levels for all subtests for that reason, and the assessment is not standardized or validated.

Use of Standardized Assessments with People with ASD and CCN

Evaluation of individuals who require alternative forms of communication, such as those with CCN or sensory disabilities, is complicated by the requirements of standardized assessments for which altering testing procedures constitutes reduced validity of such assessments (DeRuyter and Becker 1988; Flanagan and Kaufman 2009; Lund et al. in press; McDougall et al. 2012). That is, translating an exam into a student's primary language, be it Spanish, American Sign Language, or via AAC, is not permitted as a best assessment practice (Lund et al. in press). For example, standardized assessments require particular responses defined as correct responses to prompts; thus, alternative symbols may be correctly or incorrectly interpreted as correct or incorrect, depending on the examiner, which again challenges the validity of the assessment (Metz et al. 2010). Further, portions of these assessments that require written responses may be problematic when the student communicates via an AAC system that has no written component (Lund et al. in press; Metz et al. 2010). Often receptive language or nonverbal IQ tests require students to point to select responses (Ross and Cress 2006), which may be problematic for children with ASD who do not understand or use pointing. Due to these issues, Flanagan and Kaufman (2009) have recommended that subtests of standardized assessment that require oral responses not be administered to individuals who cannot speak and that results of these assessments be interpreted with caution when given to individuals who require accommodations that interfere with standardized procedures. In some cases, nonverbal intelligence tests may be viable alternatives for this population (Lund et al. in press). Considering the difficulties children with ASD and CCN have in communicating, this poses challenges for practitioners when evaluating skill levels for educational purposes (DeVeney et al. 2012).

Comprehensive Developmental and Communication Assessments

Some comprehensive developmental skills assessments may provide information regarding communication, among other skills reported. The Battelle Developmental Inventory (BDI; second ed.; Newborg 2005) and the Bayley Scales of Infant Development (Bayley-III; third ed.; Bayley 2005) are often used to identify areas of impairment related to motor and cognitive functioning and language functioning in young children (DeVeney et al. 2012). The BDI is a standardized assessment that evaluates students' performance in a range of domains, including motor, cognitive, receptive language, expressive language, social, and adaptive skills via observation or parent report. It provides composite and subscores for motor, cognitive, receptive language, expressive language, personal/social, and adaptive skills. Skills are assessed via parent report and observational probes. One that was recommended by Ganz et al. (2012) and Simpson and Ganz (2012) is the Verbal Behavior Milestones Assessment and Placement Program (VB-MAPP; Sundberg 2008). The VB-MAPP is criterion referenced and provides feedback related to milestones for typically developing individuals up to approximately 4 years. For older individuals, adaptive behavior scales may be used and often include parent, teacher, and caregiver report rather than observations or skills probes.

Using a variety of communication scales in combination with subscales of developmental assessments (e.g., BDI) may yield usable results. However, assessments that focus on communication may be particularly useful in determining clinical needs in children with ASD and CCN (DeVeney et al. 2012). The following are communication assessments that have been recommended particularly for children with ASD (Tager-Flusberg et al. 2009). The Sequenced Inventory of Communication Development-Revised (SICD; Hedrick et al. 1984) is a standardized assessment of receptive and expressive language based on parent report or observation. It is appropriate for individuals functioning around 4–48 months. The Communication and Symbolic Behavior Scales (CSBS; Wetherby and Prizant 1993) is normed and standardized and is useful for up to 36 months or within that developmental range. The CSBS evaluates rate of intentional communicative acts through play wherein the evaluator probes skills by arranging communicative temptations during naturalistic interactions. The MacArthur Communicative Development Inventory (CDI): Words and Gestures (Fenson et al. 2006) is a checklist completed by caregivers to assess vocabulary comprehension and production. It is useful in identifying number of words used by the child and understanding of adults' speech. The CDI also includes more complex language skills and may be used with individuals functioning up to about 37 months; the Words and Gestures component is designed for individuals functioning up to about 18 months developmentally. It is also available in Spanish.

Informal Evaluation Procedures

Informal, or more open-ended, evaluation procedures may be helpful in filling in information that cannot be gained through more formal measures, due to the inability to adjust procedures to accommodate AAC (DeRuyter and Becker 1988). One such technique is clinical observation, which primarily involves observing communication interactions in natural contexts and taking notes regarding the necessary communicative functions and vocabulary. Natural language samples may be collected during formal evaluation procedures or during naturalistic contexts (Tager-Flusberg et al. 2009). Further, individuals with whom the person with ASD and CCN communicates frequently, or communicative partners, should be interviewed or should participate in meetings to provide information regarding the individual's history, daily and natural communication needs, and preferences (Binger et al. 2012). *The Protocol for Culturally Inclusive Assessment of AAC* (Huer 1997) may be used to gather information, via parent interview, related to cultural issues related to communication and attitude toward AAC. Questions asked might probe parental goals for his or her child, parental priorities, typical cultural activities, familiarity, and personal communication styles. Such information may provide input for the selection of an AAC mode(s). The *PESICO Template* (Schlosser et al. 2007) also can provide information gathered informally and includes guidance for the evaluator to describe the person and problem (P), people and factors in the environment (E) related to communication, important stakeholders (S) and communicative partners, needed interventions (I), comparisons (C) between interventions and between potential interventions and doing nothing, and planned outcomes (O).

Selection of AAC Goals

Selection of goals and objective related to AAC implementation should follow directly from assessment results, including informal and observational assessments. Calculator and Black (2009) reviewed the literature on AAC practices that improve inclusion of students with severe disabilities and CCN in general education settings to compile a list of best practices, which was then validated by a panel of AAC experts. Modifications on their recommendations follow. One, communication skills should be selected related to their importance to the student; that is, those that are most needed for the student to communicate effectively in their typical settings should be prioritized. Two, skills should be selected that will prioritize the student's preferences. Three, skills should be selected that will enable the student to have more independence and choice-making opportunities, such as modifying the actions of others toward them, though this should be sensitive to the family's cultural values related to independence, dependence, and interdependence. Four, challenging behaviors should be addressed by providing the student with alternative and more desirable communication behaviors. Five, goals should reflect the need of the student to communicate across all necessary contexts, situation, and through the entire day. Six, communication goals should be related, as possible, to the learning goals in the general education setting. Seven, AAC goals should reflect needs for participation in activities with family and friends, as well as with a range of communication partners who may not be familiar with his or her communication system, including goals related to initiating interactions and spontaneous communication, versus solely responding to others' questions and prompts. Eight, skills and the AAC system selected should be based on assessment results related to previous communication skills, literacy skills, intellectual and cognitive skills, type of display, symbol comprehension, and categorization and arrangement of symbols. Nine, skills targeted should include both expressive and receptive communication.

Conclusions

Assessment of individuals with both ASD and CCN is complicated by both the lack of comprehensible speech and significant difficulties with social functioning that are common in this population. Unfortunately, few guidelines exist to provide evaluators with specific assessment tools to determine the most suitable AAC mode and properly evaluate skills in people with ASD and CCN. In particular, few assessment tools exist that are appropriate for nonspeaking adolescents and adults with ASD; most communication assessment tools are designed for young children. Thus, significant work remains in the development and widespread use of assessments in this area. Collaboration among interdisciplinary teams (see Chap. 4) is key to promoting a thorough evaluation that considers all of the strengths and needs of individuals with ASD and CCN (Batorowicz and Shepherd 2011; Dietz et al. 2012), particularly related to communication. Interdisciplinary teams should focus in particular on determining communication needs and setting AAC goal across all potential environments, individuals, and contexts.

References

Bailey, J., McComas, J., Benavidas, C., & Lovascz, C. (2002). Functional assessment in a residential setting: Identifying an effective communicative replacement response for aggressive behavior. *Journal of Developmental and Physical Disabilities, 14*, 353–369.

Batorowicz, B., & Shepherd, T. A. (2011). Teamwork in AAC: Examining clinical perceptions. *Augmentative and Alternative Communication, 27*, 16–25. doi:10.3109/07434618.2010.546809.

Bayley, N. (2005). *Bayley Scales of Infant and Toddler Development* (3rd ed.). San Antonio, TX: Pearson.

Binger, C., Ball, L., Dietz, A., Kent-Walsh, J., Lasker, J., Lund, S., …Quach, W. (2012). Personnel roles in the AAC assessment process. *Augmentative and Alternative Communication, 28*, 278–288. doi: 10.3109/07434618.2012.716079.

Bruno, J. (2006). *Test of aided-communication symbol performance*. Solana Beach, CA: Mayer-Johnson.

Calculator, S. N., & Black, T. (2009). Validation of an inventory of best practices in the provision of augmentative and alternative communication services to students with severe disabilities in general education classrooms. *American Journal of Speech-Language Pathology, 18*, 329–342.

Cannella-Malone, H., DeBar, R. M., & Sigafoos, J. (2009). An examination of preference for augmentative and alternative communication devices with two boys with significant intellectual disabilities. *Augmentative and Alternative Communication, 25*, 262–273. doi:10.3109/07434610903384511.

DeRuyter, F., & Becker, M. R. (1988). Augmentative communication: Assessment, system selection, and usage. *Journal of Head Trauma Rehabilitation, 3*, 35–44.

DeVeney, S. L., Hoffman, L., & Cress, C. J. (2012). Communication-based assessment of developmental age for young children with developmental disabilities. *Journal of Speech, Language & Hearing Research, 55*, 695–709. doi:10.1044/1092-4388(2011/10-0148).

Dietz, A., Quach, W., Lund, S. K., & McKelvey, M. (2012). AAC assessment and clinical-decision making: The impact of experience. *Augmentative and Alternative Communication, 28*, 148–159. doi:10.3109/07434618.2012.704521.

Dynavox Mayer-Johnson (1981–2009). *Picture Communication Symbols* (PCS). Retrieved from https://www.mayer-johnson.com/.

Fenson, L., Marchman, V. A., Thal, D. J., Dale, P. S., Reznick, J. S., & Bates, E. (2006). *MacArthur Communicative Development Inventories user's guide and technical manual* (2nd ed.). Baltimore, MD: Brookes.

Flanagan, D. P., & Kaufman, A. S. (2009). *Essentials of WISC-IV assessment* (2nd ed.). Hoboken, NJ: Wiley.

Flippin, M., Reszka, S., & Watson, L. R. (2010). Effectiveness of the Picture Exchange Communication System (PECS) on communication and speech for children with autism spectrum disorders: A meta-analysis. *American Journal of Speech-Language Pathology, 19*, 178–195.

Ganz, J. B., Parker, R., & Benson, J. (2009). Impact of the Picture Exchange Communication System: Effects on communication and collateral effects on maladaptive behaviors. *Augmentative and Alternative Communication, 25*, 250–261. doi:10.3109/07434610903381111.

Ganz, J. B., Simpson, R. L., & Lund, E. M. (2012). The picture exchange communication system (PECS): A promising method for improving communication skills of learners with autism spectrum disorders. *Education and Training in Autism and Developmental Disabilities, 47*, 176–186.

Heath, A. K. (2012). A meta-analysis of single-case studies on functional communication training. *Dissertation Abstracts International Section A: Humanities and Social Sciences, 73*(12). Ann Arbor, MI: ProQuest Information & Learning. UMI Number: 3524731.

Hedrick, D. L., Prather, E. M., & Tobin, A. R. (Eds.). (1984). *Sequenced Inventory of Communication Development (Rev. Ed.): Test manual*. Seattle, WA: University of Washington Press.

Heflin, J., & Alaimo, D. (2007). *Students with autism spectrum disorders: Effective instructional practices*. Upper Saddle River, NJ: Pearson and Merrill/Prentice Hall.

Huer, M. B. (1997). Culturally inclusive assessments for children using augmentative and alternative communication (AAC). *Journal of Children's Communication Development, 19*, 23–34.

Jagaroo, V., & Wilkinson, K. (2008). Further considerations of visual cognitive neuroscience in aided AAC: The potential role of motion perception systems in maximizing design display. *Augmentative and Alternative Communication, 5*, 137–144.

Light, J. (1997). "Let's go star fishing": Reflections on the contexts of language learning for children who use aided AAC. *Augmentative and Alternative Communication, 13*, 158–171. doi:10.1080/07434619712331277978.

Light, J., & McNaughton, D. (2012). Supporting the communication, language, and literacy development of children with complex communication needs: State of the science and future research priorities. *Assistive Technology, 24*, 34–44.

Lund, E. M., Miller, K. B., & Ganz, J. B. (in press). Access to assessment? Legal and practical issues regarding psychoeducational assessment in children with sensory disabilities. *Journal of Disability Policy Studies*. doi: 10.1177/1044207313478661.

McDougall, S., Vessoyan, K., & Duncan, B. (2012). Traditional versus computerized presentation and response methods on a structured AAC assessment tool. *Augmentative and Alternative Communication, 28*, 127–135. doi:10.3109/07434618.2012.677958.

McFadd, E., & Wilkinson, K. (2010). Qualitative analysis of decision making by speech-language pathologists in the design of aided visual displays. *Augmentative and Alternative Communication, 26*, 136–147. doi:10.3109/07434618.2010.481089.

Metz, K., Miller, M., & Thomas-Presswood, T. (2010). Assessing children who are deaf or hard of hearing. In D. C. Miller (Ed.), *Best practices in school neuropsychology: Guidelines for effective practice, assessment, and evidence-based intervention* (pp. 419–463). Hoboken, NJ: Wiley.

Mineo, B. A., Peischl, D., & Pennington, C. (2008). Moving targets: The effect of animation on identification of action word representations. *Augmentative and Alternative Communication, 24*, 162–173.

Mirenda, P. (2001). Autism, augmentative communication and assistive technology: What do we really know? *Focus on Autism and Other Developmental Disabilities, 16*, 141–151.

Newborg, J. (2005). *Battelle Developmental Inventory: Examiner's manual* (2nd ed.). Itasca, IL: Riverside.

Ogletree, B. (2008). The communicative context of autism. In R. Simpson & B. Myles (Eds.), *Educating children and youth with autism* (pp. 223–265). Austin, TX: Pro-Ed.

Pyramid Educational Consultants. (2013). *FAQ*. Retrieved from http://www.pecsusa.com

Ringdahl, J. E., Falcomata, T. S., Christensen, T. J., Bass-Ringdahl, S. M., Lentz, A., Dutt, A., & Schuh-Claus, J. (2009). Evaluation of a pre-treatment assessment to select mand topographies for functional communication training. *Research in Developmental Disabilities, 30*, 330–341. doi: 2048/10.1016/j.ridd.2008.06.002.

Ross, B., & Cress, C. J. (2006). Comparison of standardized assessments for cognitive and receptive communication skills in young children with complex communication needs. *Augmentative and Alternative Communication, 22*, 100–111. doi:10.1080/07434610500389629.

Schlosser, R. W., Koul, R., & Costello, J. (2007). Asking well-built questions for evidence-based practice in augmentative and alternative communication. *Journal of Communication Disorders, 40*, 225–238.

Sigafoos, J., Green, V. A., Payne, D., Son, S., O'Reilly, M., & Lancioni, G. E. (2009). A comparison of picture exchange and speech-generating devices: Acquisition, preference, and effects on social interaction. *Augmentative and Alternative Communication, 25*, 99–109. doi:10.1080/07434610902739959.

Simpson, R. L., & Ganz, J. B. (2012). The picture exchange communication system (PECS). In P. Prelock & R. McCauley (Eds.), *Treatment of autism spectrum disorders: Evidence-based intervention strategies for communication & social interaction* (pp. 255–280). Baltimore: Paul H Brookes.

Stafford, A., Alberto, P., Fredrick, L., Heflin, L., & Heller, K. (2002). Preference variability and the instruction of choice making with students with severe intellectual disabilities. *Education and Training in Mental Retardation and Developmental Disabilities, 37*, 70–88.

Sundberg, M. L. (2008). VB-MAPP Verbal Behavior Milestones Assessment and Placement Program: A language and social skills assessment program for children with autism or other developmental disabilities: Guide. Concord, CA: AVB Press.

Tager-Flusberg, H., Rogers, S., Cooper, J., Landa, R., Lord, C., Paul, R., … Yoder, P. (2009). Defining spoken language benchmarks and selecting measures of expressive language development for young children with autism spectrum disorders. *Journal of Speech, Language, and Hearing Research, 52,* 643–652. doi: 10.1044/1092-4388(2009/08-0136).

van der Meer, L., Sigafoos, J., O'Reilly, M. F., & Lancioni, G. E. (2011). Assessing preferences for AAC options in communication interventions for individuals with developmental disabilities: A review of the literature. *Research in Developmental Disabilities, 32,* 1422–1431.

Von Tetzchner, S., & Martinsen, H. (1992). *Introduction to symbolic and augmentative communication.* San Diego, CA: Singular Publishing.

Wetherby, A. M., & Prizant, B. M. (1993). *Communication and Symbolic Behavior Scales (Normed ed.): Manual.* Baltimore, MD: Brookes.

Winborn-Kemmerer, L., Wacker, D. P., & Harding, J. (2010). Analysis of mand selection across different stimulus conditions. *Education and Treatment of Children, 33,* 49–64.

Chapter 4
Interdisciplinary Issues and Collaboration in Assessment and Treatment

Collaboration across a range of disciplines and stakeholders is central to successful implementation of aided AAC programming. People with ASD and CCN are typically served by a wide range of professionals, such as school psychologists, speech-language pathologists (SLPs), teachers, and paraprofessionals (i.e., school aides). Because communication skills are needed in every setting, communication, careful planning, and cooperation across these professionals and with family members are critical to ensure that all stakeholders are implementing AAC. Collaboration is particularly important given the varied areas of expertise across disciplines. For example, SLPs have reported that they have little knowledge or skills in providing reading and writing instruction to people who use AAC (Simpson et al. 1998); thus, educators and speech-language professionals must work together to address such issues in the students they share. Further, time to collaborate is typically greatly needed and often overlooked when considering collaboration needs between general and special educators, between educators and related service providers, and between professionals and family members (Calculator and Black 2009). Input from all stakeholders, including family members and the person with CCN, related to multimodal AAC options and preferences should be investigated. Roles and needs of each of these groups are discussed below.

Beyond distinct roles, skills in collaboration are needed to successfully work in teams to meet the needs of individuals with ASD and CCN (Kent-Walsh et al. 2008). All team members should attend professional development and engage in self-teaching activities to learn how to collaborate and meet the needs of children with CCN in their classrooms (Fallon and Katz 2008). First, collaboration skills are one key to successful interdisciplinary teamwork (Kent-Walsh et al. 2008; Soto et al. 2001). Collaboration includes having effective communication among the team, working toward common goals for the student, respecting input from all stakeholders, determining roles and responsibilities while maintaining some flexibility around those roles, meeting regularly, efficiency in team meetings, and school–family collaboration (Fallon and Katz 2008; McSheehan et al. 2006; Soto et al. 2001). Second, teams must determine how students will use AAC to access general education

J.B. Ganz, *Aided Augmentative Communication for Individuals with Autism Spectrum Disorders*, Autism and Child Psychopathology Series, DOI 10.1007/978-1-4939-0814-1_4,
© Springer Science+Business Media New York 2014

curriculum (Soto et al. 2001). This should include, for example, literacy instruction for students with CCN, access of the general education curriculum via AAC, and instructional practices in AAC (McSheehan et al. 2006). Team members must have an understanding of the typical curriculum (Soto et al. 2001). Third, team members, particularly those who are providing direct services to the individual with CCN, must have a basic understanding and abilities regarding the student's AAC system operation, maintenance, and programming (Soto et al. 2001). All members need to have basic skills in implementing interventions to promote the student's use of the AAC device(s), including adding needed vocabulary. At the least, each team member who provides direct services should have knowledge of resources that may be used for tech support in such instances. Beyond collaboration skills, teams who work with people with CCN should also have training in how to promote participation of students with CCN in their classrooms, how to support these students to maximize their participation (Kent-Walsh et al. 2008; McSheehan et al. 2006).

Family Role and Preference of People with ASD in Selecting and Implementing AAC

Family members, as primary communicative partners, are perhaps the most important members of interdisciplinary AAC teams. Buy-in of family member for a given AAC system is needed if individuals with ASD and CCN are to generalize the use of AAC into their homes and communities (Calculator and Black 2009). Considerations of preferences of family members of and individuals with ASD are key to preventing abandonment of the system or device (Angelo 2000; Calculator and Black 2009). Integration of AAC may be challenging to family members, who are often already quite challenged by caring for their family member who has ASD and CCN, particularly when AAC systems do not meet their needs or expectations (Delarosa et al. 2012) or are deemed by them to be impractical (Mirenda 2003). When professionals collaborate with family members to implement AAC, particularly high-tech AAC, the amount of time needed to learn to use such systems and to program them may be of significant concern; complex technologies may limit the addition of new vocabulary and limit the individuals progress unless easy to update apps are available (i.e., "just-in-time" technology; Light and McNaughton 2012). Further, family member may need assistance in identifying and planning for opportunities for individuals with ASD and CCN to communicate (Sigafoos 1999). More information regarding working directly with family members is provided in Chap. 6.

A potential tool to assist in working with families, the Family Impact of Assistive Technology Scale for Augmentative and Alternative Communication (FIATS-AAC), was developed to evaluate the impact of AAC implementation on families of children who use AAC via a Likert scale parent report tool (Delarosa et al. 2012). Areas evaluated are derived from the World Health Organization's (WHO 2007) conceptual framework for the International Classification of Functioning, Disability, and

Health for Children and Youth (ICF-CY), which emphasizes physical functioning (body structure and function), daily tasks in which the child is engaged (activities), and his or her engagement in typical life events (participation). Specifically, the FIATS-AAC has the following preliminary domains: family roles in caregiving, parental concerns regarding safety, social interaction, conversation, parental health and well-being, parent level of effort in caring for their child, child level of control over his or her activities, appropriateness of child behavior, success at school, need for supervision from family members, parental need for respite and relief, child level of contentment, child ability to engage in activities autonomously, and level of family financial difficulties (Delarosa et al. 2012). The FIATS-AAC was determined to have good internal consistency and test–retest reliability (i.e., when repeated several weeks after the first administration, the scores were similar to the first administration) (Delarosa et al. 2012). While the FIATS-AAC does not appear to be available for purchase at this time, the tool appears to give some recommendations for important areas of consideration when determining the suitability of a particular AAC system for a family.

Although, given the common communication deficits, it may be difficult to determine the preferences related to AAC mode of an individual with ASD and CCN, some researchers have made attempts to do so (van der Meer et al. 2011). Preference is typically assessed by placing two or more AAC modes in front of the participant and asking him or her to tell the interventionist what he or she wanted by pointing or taking that device; the researchers presumed that the mode used most often was the preferred mode (Cannella-Malone et al. 2009; van der Meer et al. 2011). In some cases, this selection was made prior to instruction (van der Meer et al. 2012). More often, preferences were assessed following evidence that the individual was able to correctly match items requested via icons with the actual items (Cannella-Malone et al. 2009). Typically, these AAC preference assessments take place following at least a small amount of instruction in the use of each system (Cannella-Malone et al. 2009), presumably to ensure that choices are made related to preference versus familiarity with or mastery of one particular system. At times, preference may need to be reevaluated to determine if preference has changed (Stafford et al. 2002). Unfortunately, research in the area of preference of AAC devices by people with CCN is not yet well developed, and it is unclear what variables factor into individuals' choices (van der Meer et al. 2011). Further information regarding assessment of AAC preference of family members and individuals with ASD and CCN is provided in Chap. 3.

Role of School Psychologists

School psychologists and diagnosticians have an important role related to adequate and accurate assessment of students with ASD and CCN. They are likely to play a role both in assessment for individuals who use AAC and in assisting in selection of an AAC system or device (Parette and Marr 1997). Parette and Marr provide recommendations to school psychologists to consider when assisting in selection of AAC systems. These recommendations include consideration of the child, including appropriate individualization of assessment procedures to accommodate for AAC, observations of the student in a variety of contexts, and consideration of the student's preferences. AAC considerations include identification of resources to aid in the selection of AAC, information about the pros and cons of the devices or systems being considered, good match between the student's characteristics and the AAC system, and costs of the device and its maintenance, including insurance considerations. Further, Parette and Marr suggest consideration of the family's needs, such as those related to their expectation related to assessment, their concerns for their child, inclusion of them as partners in the assessment and selection process, and the family's prior experience with assistive technology. Finally, Parette and Marr recommend that school psychologists consider cultural expectations, such as the family's personal values and beliefs, the family's attitude about disabilities, extended family that may need to be involved in the process, communication between the family and professionals, and cultural issues or expectations related to AAC. Assessments of students with ASD and CCN and selection of AAC systems are discussed more thoroughly in Chap. 3.

Role of Speech-Language Pathologists

SLPs may have a number of roles on AAC teams. To some degree, their roles may vary depending on their levels of knowledge, skill, and experience in AAC (Beukelman et al. 2008; Hustad et al. 2008). That is, AAC experts may have significant expertise and may fill all the roles that follow or may serve as consultants. SLPs in schools or other integrated practices may provide a range of SLP services and have some knowledge related to AAC and may be primarily responsible for providing direct services. SLPs with little knowledge of AAC may serve as referrers to other service providers or may call in experts to assist with AAC implementation (Beukelman et al. 2008; Binger et al. 2012; Hustad et al. 2008).

Specific tasks and roles in which each of the above may be involved include the following. For one, SLPs may be the first to recognize the need for AAC and play a role in referring the individual for further evaluation by an AAC expert (Binger et al. 2012). Two, SLPs play a role in assessment and selection of goals and objectives. They may select and implement communication assessments (Beukelman et al. 2008; Grether and Sickman 2008). Relatedly, SLPs may be instrumental in the identification of general education and individualized language and literacy objectives (Grether and Sickman 2008). Further, SLPs often serve in the role of finding and selecting AAC devices (Beukelman et al. 2008; Binger et al. 2012) and finding funding for high-tech devices (Dietz et al. 2012). Communication assessment and selection of AAC mode are discussed in detail in Chap. 3.

Three, SLPs often share the role of implementation of AAC with educators. Often, speech services are provided via pull-out sessions; however, more integrated approaches to promoting communication and AAC use within natural settings are warranted (Calculator and Black 2009); particularly because the purpose of AAC is to enhance functional communication, not use of communication in isolation. SLPs may be particularly helpful in preparing curricular materials, such as communication boards to support literacy learning (Grether and Sickman 2008) and in implementation of positive behavior supports (Bopp et al. 2004). This may include selecting and making educational accommodations and modifications, such as increasing the efficiency of answering questions by requiring multiple choice answers instead of short answer test questions (Grether and Sickman 2008). Relatedly, SLPs who have expertise in implementation of AAC may be responsible for providing staff development in AAC implementation and language and literacy instruction for family members, for classmates, and for other professionals who work directly with individuals with ASD and CCN (Grether and Sickman 2008).

Four, SLPs should share the role of progress monitoring with educators (Grether and Sickman 2008). However, beyond whether or not AAC may be used successfully in controlled speech sessions, SLPs should also collect data on the use of AAC in natural contexts to determining whether or not people with ASD and CCN are able to communicate in typical settings (Calculator and Black 2009). Data on the use of AAC and mastery of related communication goals should be collected regularly and SLPs should regularly review these data to determine the effectiveness of the AAC system, make modifications, add vocabulary, revise goals, and determine professional development needs. This process should be ongoing to insure that needed modifications in AAC mode and vocabulary are made to meet the communication needs of students with ASD and CCN across all settings and contexts (Grether and Sickman 2008).

Roles of Educators, Paraprofessionals, and Daily Service Providers

Educators, including paraprofessionals and other assistants, have the primary role for implementing AAC-based interventions across school contexts. Because they, along with parents, are often the most frequent communicative partners, they are often responsible for maintaining the AAC device/system, meeting the individual's needs related to AAC, and encouraging AAC use (Binger et al. 2012). Further, supervising teachers play a significant role in training and monitoring of paraprofessionals, or aides, who often spend more time with individuals with ASD and CCN in school than certified teachers do (Binger et al. 2010). Intervention is covered in detail in Chaps. 5 and 6.

Classroom teachers and paraprofessionals play a primary role in progress monitoring (Grether and Sickman 2008). Teachers and paraprofessionals who work with the individual who uses AAC should regularly collect data on the person's progress in effectively using the system, progress on related goals, use related to general education curricula, use across various contexts and settings, use with varied communication partners and peers, use across the day (Calculator and Black 2009).

Further, it is crucial that educators collect data on AAC and communication across all possible natural contexts and settings, including in the home and community when possible, to assess the communication abilities of people with ASD and CCN in typical contexts (Calculator and Black 2009).

Educators also play a key role in the integration of children with CCN into classrooms, including general education settings (Finke et al. 2009). Children with significant disabilities who are frequently included in general education settings are often rejected by their peers and socially isolated (Finke et al. 2009; McDougall et al. 2004). This can be particularly true for students with disabilities that negatively impact their ability to communicate with peers effectively (Beck et al. 2010). While schools cannot control outside factors, such as attitudes imparted by parents, gender, and prior negative experiences, all of which have been shown to impact attitudes of peers (McDougall et al. 2004), there are a number of things educators can do to promote successful inclusion of people with ASD and CCN in general education settings.

In particular, the following factors have been found to correlate with positive attitudes of peers about their classmates with disabilities or have been recommended by experts in AAC (Calculator and Black 2009; McDougall et al. 2004). One, AAC programming must be integrated into all other educational planning (Calculator and Black 2009). That is, goals should not be simply be written for AAC communication, but the entire schedule must be investigated to determine how and when communication can be supported with the use of AAC, across all school subjects and contexts. AAC should be seen as not a goal in and of itself but as a means via which people with ASD and CCN can be supported members of the school community (Calculator and Black 2009). Such an integrated approach must involve collaboration of all relevant team members. For example, in providing literacy instruction to people with ASD and CCN, expertise from general and special educators with knowledge of literacy instruction and expertise from SLPs and AAC specialists will probably be needed (Fallon and Katz 2008).

Two, promotion of friendship and cooperation is one means of successfully integrating people with ASD and CCN into general education settings. School environments that promote cooperative activities and learning for all versus competitive activities have been associated with more positive attitudes toward peers with disabilities (McDougall et al. 2004). AAC skills specifically targeting development of friendships should be included in AAC program planning (Calculator and Black 2009). However, a balance should be realized between supporting the student and providing room for friendships to develop without obtrusive adult supports (Soto et al. 2001).

Three, peers who are more familiar with and have more experience with people who use AAC have better attitudes toward them (Beck et al. 2010). Thus, students with ASD and CCN should be seen as full members of the classroom. That is, teachers and others should communicate that such students have the same role and participation expectations as all students (McSheehan et al. 2006). Such expectations can be demonstrated by ensuring that the student has an assigned place in the classroom, including him or her in routines, including him or her in cooperative group activities, and being called on and responding in class (Finke et al. 2009; McSheehan et al. 2006; Soto et al. 2001).

Four, for older children and adults, positive attitudes have been found to be related to the level of technology used by the person with CCN (Gorenflo and Gorenflo 1994; Lilienfeld and Alant 2005); that is, newer and higher tech systems have been found to be viewed more favorably by peers. Additionally, peers may be taught how the system works and how they can encourage interactions (Soto et al. 2001). Five, voice output appears to have a positive impact on peer attitudes toward children who use AAC (Gorenflo and Gorenflo 1994). Thus, higher-tech devices may be good options if a clear preference for a device is not otherwise apparent. Six, peer training to encourage and teach skills related to interacting via AAC appears to have a positive effect on outcomes (Lilienfeld and Alant 2005). This may include instruction in conversational turn-taking, allowing the person with CCN to initiate interactions, listening, and maintaining interactions (Grether and Sickman 2008). For further and more descriptive ideas on promoting peer-mediated interventions involving AAC, see Chap. 6.

Conclusions

In conclusion, it is critical that AAC interventions are not implemented in isolation. Implementing AAC in one setting without consideration of the needs and preferences of all stakeholders is one factor in the likelihood of AAC abandonment (Angelo 2000). One way to ensure that AAC is generalized across settings, and thus serves as a truly functional communication system, is by working collaboratively across fields and with family members, learning skills in implementing AAC, and ensuring support for and oversight of the roles of all individuals involved.

References

Angelo, D. H. (2000). Impact of augmentative and alternative communication devices on families. *Augmentative and Alternative Communication, 16*, 37–47.

Beck, A. R., Thompson, J. R., Kosuwan, K., & Prochnow, J. M. (2010). The development and utilization of a scale to measure adolescents' attitudes toward peers who use augmentative and alternative communication (AAC) devices. *Journal of Speech, Language, and Hearing Research, 53*, 572–587.

Beukelman, D. R., Ball, L. J., & Fager, S. (2008). An AAC personnel framework: Adults with acquired complex communication needs. *Augmentative and Alternative Communication, 24*, 255–267. doi:10.1080/07434610802388477.

Binger, C., Ball, L., Dietz, A., Kent-Walsh, J., Lasker, J., Lund, S., & Quach, W. (2012). Personnel roles in the AAC assessment process. *Augmentative and Alternative Communication, 28*, 278–288. doi:10.3109/07434618.2012.716079.

Binger, C., Kent-Walsh, J., Ewing, C., & Taylor, S. (2010). Teaching educational assistants to facilitate the multisymbol message productions of young students who require augmentative and alternative communication. *American Journal of Speech-Language Pathology, 19*, 108–120. doi:10.1044/1058-0360(2009/09-0015).

Bopp, K. D., Brown, K. E., & Mirenda, P. (2004). Speech-language pathologists' roles in the delivery of positive behavior support for individuals with developmental disabilities. *American Journal of Speech-Language Pathology, 13*, 5–19.

Calculator, S. N., & Black, T. (2009). Validation of an inventory of best practices in the provision of augmentative and alternative communication services to students with severe disabilities in general education classrooms. *American Journal of Speech-Language Pathology, 18*, 329–342.

Cannella-Malone, H., DeBar, R. M., & Sigafoos, J. (2009). An examination of preference for augmentative and alternative communication devices with two boys with significant intellectual disabilities. *Augmentative and Alternative Communication, 25*, 262–273. doi:10.3109/07434610903384511.

Delarosa, E., Horner, S., Eisenberg, C., Ball, L., Renzoni, A. M., & Ryan, S. E. (2012). Family impact of assistive technology scale: Development of a measurement scale for parents of children with complex communication needs. *Augmentative and Alternative Communication, 28*, 171–180. doi:10.3109/07434618.2012.704525.

Dietz, A., Quach, W., Lund, S. K., & McKelvey, M. (2012). AAC assessment and clinical-decision making: The impact of experience. *Augmentative and Alternative Communication, 28*, 148–159. doi:10.3109/07434618.2012.704521.

Fallon, K. A., & Katz, L. A. (2008). Augmentative and alternative communication and literacy teams: Facing the challenges, forging ahead. *Seminars in Speech & Language, 29*, 112–119.

Finke, E. H., McNaughton, D. B., & Drager, K. D. R. (2009). "All children can and should have the opportunity to learn": General education teachers' perspectives on including children with autism spectrum disorder who require AAC. *Augmentative and Alternative Communication, 25*, 110–122. doi:10.1080/07434610902886206.

Gorenflo, C. W., & Gorenflo, D. W. (1994). Effects of synthetic voice output attitudes toward the augmented communicator. *Journal of Speech and Hearing Research, 37*, 64–68.

Grether, S. M., & Sickman, L. S. (2008). AAC and RTI: Building classroom-based strategies for every child in the classroom. *Seminars in Speech and Language, 29*, 155–163. doi:10.1055/s-2008-1079129.

Hustad, K. C., Keppner, K., Schanz, A., & Berg, A. (2008). Augmentative and alternative communication for preschool children: Intervention goals and use of technology. *Seminars in Speech and Language, 29*, 83–91. doi:10.1055/s-2008-1080754.

Kent-Walsh, J., Stark, C., & Binger, C. (2008). Tales from school trenches: AAC service-delivery and professional expertise. *Seminars in Speech and Language, 29*, 146–154. doi:10.1055/s-2008-1079128.

Light, J., & McNaughton, D. (2012). Supporting the communication, language, and literacy development of children with complex communication needs: State of the science and future research priorities. *Assistive Technology, 24*, 34–44.

Lilienfeld, M., & Alant, E. (2005). The social interaction of an adolescent who uses AAC: The evaluation of a peer-training program. *Augmentative and Alternative Communication, 21*, 278–294. doi:10.1080/07434610500103467.

McDougall, J., Dewit, D. J., King, G., Mille, L. T., & Killip, S. (2004). High school-aged youths' attitudes toward their peers with disabilities: The role of school and student interpersonal factors. *International Journal of Disability, Development & Education, 51*, 287–313. doi:10.1080/1034912042000259242.

McSheehan, M., Sonnenmeier, R. M., Jorgensen, C. M., & Turner, K. (2006). Beyond communication access: Promoting learning of the general education curriculum by students with significant disabilities. *Topics in Language Disorders, 26*, 266–290.

Mirenda, P. (2003). Toward functional augmentative and alternative communication for students with autism: Manual signs, graphic symbols, and voice output communication aids. *Language, Speech, and Hearing Services in Schools, 34*, 203–216.

Parette, H. P., & Marr, D. D. (1997). Assisting children and families who use augmentative and alternative communication (AAC) devices: Best practices for school psychologists. *Psychology in the Schools, 34*, 337–346.

Sigafoos, J. (1999). Creating opportunities for augmentative and alternative communication: Strategies for involving people with developmental disabilities. *Augmentative and Alternative Communication, 15*, 183–190.

Simpson, K., Beukelman, D., & Bird, A. (1998). Survey of school speech and language service provision to students with severe communication impairments in Nebraska. *Augmentative and Alternative Communication, 14*, 212–221.

Soto, G., Müller, E., Hunt, P., & Goetz, L. (2001). Professional skills for serving students who use AAC in general education classrooms: A team perspective. *Language, Speech, and Hearing Services in Schools, 32*, 51–56.

Stafford, A., Alberto, P., Fredrick, L., Heflin, L., & Heller, K. (2002). Preference variability and the instruction of choice making with students with severe intellectual disabilities. *Education and Training in Mental Retardation and Developmental Disabilities, 37*, 70–88.

van der Meer, L., Sigafoos, J., O'Reilly, M. F., & Lancioni, G. E. (2011). Assessing preferences for AAC options in communication interventions for individuals with developmental disabilities: A review of the literature. *Research in Developmental Disabilities, 32*, 1422–1431.

van der Meer, L., Sutherland, D., O'Reilly, M. F., Lancioni, G. E., & Sigafoos, J. (2012). A further comparison of manual signing, picture exchange, and speech-generating devices as communication modes for children with autism spectrum disorders. *Research in Autism Spectrum Disorders, 6*, 1247–1257.

World Health Organization (WHO). (2007). *ICF-CY, International Classification of Functioning, Disability, and Health: Children & Youth version*. Geneva: World Health Organization.

Part II
Interventions and Techniques to Provide Aided AAC for People with ASD

Chapter 5
Naturalistic Aided AAC Instruction

Jennifer B. Ganz and Ee Rea Hong

Scenario

Scotty, a 10-year old with ASD and CCN, had acquired the use of his tablet computer-based SGD app to make requests for over 20 food items and toys. His behavioral therapist, Ella, sitting across the kitchen table from Scotty, held up a rainmaker toy, and Scotty spontaneously pushed the button that had the toy's picture. The app played the recording of a male voice saying "rainmaker," and Ella handed him the toy, which Scotty held close to his ear as he listened to the beads drop. After about 10 s, said, "my turn," and took the rainmaker back. Scotty immediately tapped the picture of the rainmaker on his app again, repeating the sequence. After a few turns, while Scotty was listening to the beads, Ella stopped to jot down data. She was pleased with his progress; however, Ella quickly noted that he never spontaneously asked for the rainmaker in other rooms, with other therapists, or if there were other objects on the table, even though, when offered a choice among multiple objects, Scotty chose the rainmaker almost every time and would seek it out whenever they sat at the kitchen table where they practiced using his communication app. One day, she put his tablet computer on the table near him, showed him a photo of the rainmaker from a slightly different angle than the photo on his app, and asked him, "what's that?" Scotty leaned close to and peered at the picture but did not answer her question. Over coffee with another teacher, Ella, clearly frustrated, exclaimed, "it's like he's stuck!" Her colleague said, "no, you just need a plan to teach him, strategically, to communicate in a variety of contexts and for a variety of communicative purposes."

(continued)

J.B. Ganz, *Aided Augmentative Communication for Individuals with Autism Spectrum Disorders*, Autism and Child Psychopathology Series, DOI 10.1007/978-1-4939-0814-1_5, © Springer Science+Business Media New York 2014

(continued)

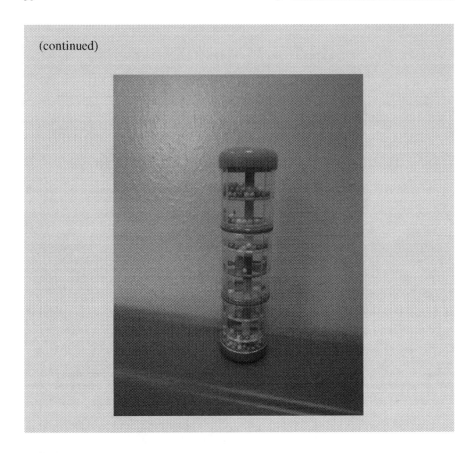

Introduction

Individuals with ASD who use AAC are often isolated from others, both as a function of the disability itself and as a function of the difficulty communicating via conventional means (Veness et al. 2012). That is, individuals who use AAC may be more passive in conversations, may communicate for only a few purposes, may communicate less frequently than peers, and may have increased rates of communication breakdowns (King and Fahsl 2012). While AAC instruction in structured settings, such as school and clinical environments, is critical, it is also critical that individuals with CCN learn to use AAC in all settings and contexts (Calculator 1999). Thus, this chapter is aimed at providing information regarding the implementation of AAC instruction within natural contexts, including providing background information, a summary of implementation, a review of research, and conclusions.

Hart and Risley's (1978, 1980, 1989, 1992, 2003) early investigations of the impact of parental interactions with their children had a number of findings that are relevant to naturalistic instruction and that, in fact, led to their development of a model called incidental teaching. Following years of observations of young children and their parents in their homes, Hart and Risley (1992) found that particular parent interaction style and behavior factors were related to child outcomes in IQ and language use. In particular, the amount of language parents modeled for and feedback given to their children and the quality of the interactions were correlated with child IQ.

The language models and feedback included several components that correlated with higher IQs in the children (Hart and Risley 1992). One, parents stayed in close proximity for a greater extent of time, which gave them more opportunities to provide language models and respond to their children's initiations. Two, parents joined in activities and communications in which the children were engaging in. That is, incidental teaching opportunities naturally became available when parents commented on what their children were doing and responded to their children's utterances. Three, parents modeled a variety of different words and concepts. This included interactions related to objects in the children's presence, often arranged so by the parents to provide opportunities to talk about new words and concepts and narrating what the children were doing.

Quality of interactions also had several key components that correlated with higher IQs in the children (Hart and Risley 1992). One, parents frequently repeated and expanded on what their children said. That is, they were responsive to children's initiations in a number of ways. They sometimes repeated what their children said to confirm their understanding, particularly when the children's language was difficult to understand. They also frequently expanded on what their children said, thereby adding and modeling new content. Two, parents often asked their children questions to encourage them to take a turn in conversation. This occurred even before the children started talking. Three, parents infrequently used prohibitions. That is, instead of providing negative feedback, they often redirected children to age-appropriate materials rather than restricting, correcting, or criticizing, which could lead to less exploration.

As a result of their work recording language experiences in young children, Hart and Risley (2003) have made several suggestions regarding providing instruction to children who have had limited language experiences during early language development. Granted, these recommendations were generally for typically developing children; however, given the issues surrounding generalization of skills to untrained contexts for people with ASD, that incidental teaching has some evidence of effectiveness with children with ASD (Charlop-Christy and Carpenter 2000; McGee and Daly 2007; McGee et al. 1999; Miranda-Linne and Melin 1992) when used for verbal language instruction naturalistic instruction, and that naturalistic AAC instruction (discussed below) has some research support, incidental teaching and other naturalistic instructional approaches applied to AAC instruction warrant consideration.

According to Hart and Risley (1978), there are three main phases to incidental teaching. One, the child initiates an interaction (Hart and Risley 1978). Typically developing children may do this naturally and through speech. Individuals with

ASD and CCN may not yet have the AAC skills to initiate through use of the AAC device and may, due to social deficits (Mundy et al. 1986), initiate social interactions less frequently than their peers do. Thus, when using incidental teaching with people with ASD, the communicative partner must prepare the environment so that there are objects and activities that will likely motivate the individual with ASD to initiate an interaction with a person or object. Further, the communicative partner focuses his or her attention on the person using AAC, waiting with an expectant look. This will be described in more detail in later sections. Two, there is a consequence to the child's initiation that promotes language use (Hart and Risley 1978). This consequence should include an elaboration of what the child said or did. For example, such consequences may include labeling an item the child touches, asking a question for clarification or to extend the vocabulary used in the exchange, modeling the use of a descriptor (e.g., color, shape, texture), repeating the child's language use with a slightly expanded sentence, redirecting to another subject or object, or prompting the child to use specific words (e.g., physically assisting the child in selecting the correct icons on her AAC device). Three, the communicative partner ends the exchange on a positive note (Hart and Risley 1978). For example, if the child does not respond to prompts and cues for elaboration, the communicative partner may back down to a simpler form or function of communication, provide praise, and then end the exchange. Prohibitions and criticism are not used.

Naturalistic Instruction and AAC

Various approaches have been developed to provide instruction or intervention in natural and varied contexts for individuals who use AAC. These interventions fall under a variety of names, but share a number of components, particularly the focus on naturalistic instruction in the use of functional communication skills via AAC. Naturalistic interventions, sometimes called milieu teaching or incidental teaching, with AAC may involve setting up numerous communication opportunities, engaging in play routines, pausing in those routines to encourage a communicative act, and using least-to-most prompting sequences to teach the participant to use the photo exchange or other AAC system (Ogletree et al. 2012). Aided language stimulation is a naturalistic, supportive approach to improving communication in children with language delays (Jonsson et al. 2011). Primary techniques implemented during aided language stimulation include selecting AAC symbols while pairing selections with verbal models, demonstrating various syntactic and semantic combinations (Drager et al. 2006). Aided AAC modeling, similar to aided language stimulation, generally involves speaking while selecting or pointing to the relevant symbols on the individuals, AAC device (Binger and Light 2007). The System for Augmenting Language includes specific intervention components. These include using a speech-generating device, naturalistic communication opportunities, providing feedback for the child's communicative attempts, expanding vocabulary, and giving items to the child (Sevcik et al. 1995). The stress on using an SGD is due to the ability of such devices to be used to get the attention of communicative partners in typical interactions without requiring them to visually attend to the AAC device, as would be required with a picture point system (Drager et al. 2006). Natural aided language is another name for AAC modeling and involves, in addition to many of the afore-mentioned techniques, placing communication books or boards around the setting to encourage opportunities to use language throughout the day (Drager et al. 2006; Romski et al. 1996).

While naturalistic aided AAC interventions fall under a range of names, they generally share the following key components and foci, which are fairly similar to the components of incidental teaching (Hart and Risley 1978). One, naturalistic AAC interventions are implemented in the settings in which AAC-based communi-cation is expected to be used (Light 1997; Ogletree et al. 2012). Generalization of skills across settings is targeted early in the process rather than by providing inten-sive instruction in contrived circumstances. Two, natural interventions involving the implementation of aided AAC interventions include modeling of AAC use by instructors, similar to the way typically developing children learn to speak, in part, by hearing repeated models (Binger and Light 2007). Three, naturalistic AAC inter-ventions involve expanding and scaffolding based on current verbal, nonverbal, and AAC-based communication skills, taking what the person already knows a step fur-ther. Four, these interventions involve implementation of direct instruction via behavioral techniques, such as time delay, positive reinforcement, and prompting (Reichle et al. 2002). The basis for new learning typically involves starting with the skills the individual already has and building on those skills. Although direct instruc-tion of skills is given less emphasis in naturalistic interventions for typically devel-oping children and people with disabilities other than ASD, behavioral interventions are by far the most research-supported interventions for people with ASD (Eldevik et al. 2009; Howlin et al. 2009; Campbell 2003), and individuals with ASD typically do not learn as much from simply being exposed to new information without direct intervention (MacDuff et al. 2001). Thus, naturalistic interventions for AAC for this population must combine both typical naturalistic approaches (Hart and Risley 1978) with behavioral techniques to teach new skills. Five, the natural communica-tion partners are usually key interventionists. This often includes parents and peers (King and Fahsl 2012; Sevcik et al. 1995). The first four of these components are described more thoroughly below. Component five is covered in Chap. 6 on parent, caregiver, and peer-mediated interventions. Figure 5.1 provides a graphic organizer highlighting naturalistic AAC components and theoretical background.

Implementation in Natural Settings and Contexts

A primary component of naturalistic instruction in AAC is that it takes place in natural environments, with typically available materials, with all possible potential communicative partners, and within regular routines (Light 1997; Sevcik et al. 1995). That is, communicative partners, such as teachers, speech-language patholo-gists, and educational aides, should aim to incorporate instruction in how to use AAC within regular activities versus working one-on-one in a therapy room or at a

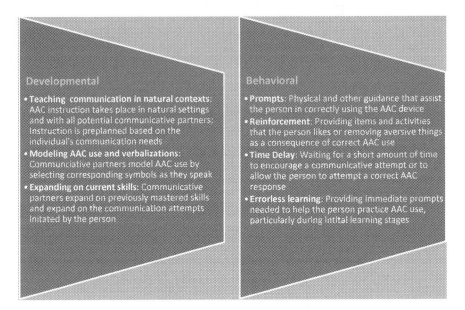

Developmental

• **Teaching communication in natural contexts:** AAC instruction takes place in natural settings and with all potential communicative partners; instruction is preplanned based on the individual's communication needs

• **Modeling AAC use and verbalizations:** Communicative partners model AAC use by selecting corresponding symbols as they speak

• **Expanding on current skills:** Communicative partners expand on previously mastered skills and expand on the communication attempts initiated by the person

Behavioral

• **Prompts:** Physical and other guidance that assist the person in correctly using the AAC device

• **Reinforcement:** Providing items and activities that the person likes or removing aversive things as a consequence of correct AAC use

• **Time Delay:** Waiting for a short amount of time to encourage a communicative attempt or to allow the person to attempt a correct AAC response

• **Errorless learning:** Providing immediate prompts needed to help the person practice AAC use, particularly during initial learning stages

Fig. 5.1 Key components of naturalistic aided AAC instruction

table in the corner of the room. To ensure generalization occurs, instruction should be planned for and strategically implemented in all possible settings, targeting multiple social contexts for intervention (Light et al. 1999). Naturalistic instruction is more than simply taking advantage of teachable moments, however. Communicative partners plan for and set up communication opportunities (Cosbey and Johnston 2006). These opportunities should involve materials and routines in which the individual with CCN engages readily, such as reinforcing objects and activities and routines that the individual engages in without significant prompting.

Wetherby and Prutting (1984) provide a number of communicative temptations that can be used to encourage opportunities to teach new communication skills. These include joining the person in an activity and having another person come take key items and walk away, using an interactive toy with the child then pausing or turning it off, holding a piece of food the person likes out to him or her and waiting for a response, spilling messy substances near the person in the middle of an activity, putting preferred items in containers that the person cannot open, reading or looking through a book or magazine with the person, and removing items that are necessary for a particular routine or activity and waiting for the person to notice. Additional communicative temptations for older individuals may involve interrupting routines by standing in the way or removing key items needed for their completion (e.g., toothbrush), putting needed or preferred items on a shelf that is in view, but cannot be reached without a step stool, or handing the person the incorrect items to complete a task or activity. Educators and communicative partners can determine other ways to set up communicative temptations, by taking notes on the typical daily routine and determining needed communication functions and vocabulary or potential ways to sabotage or interrupt typical routines and activities.

> **Scenario**
>
> Drawing from Scotty's IEP and as a result of listing his daily activities and corresponding communication needs, Ella decided to focus on, among others, the following communication objectives and initial contexts in which to target them:
>
> - Requesting help (Contexts: Computer does not work, opening containers in which his preferred items are stored and that he cannot open independently, putting on his helmet to ride his bike)
> - Labeling items (Contexts: In any setting, responding to questions about items in his environment, beginning with reinforcing items and preferred foods)
>
> Ella went through his afternoon and evening activities at home with his mother and together, they listed all of the things Scotty chose to use or play with. For each room or activity, Ella programed a page on the communication app with all of the vocabulary symbols, a HELP symbol, and a WHAT'S-THAT symbol.
>
> The first day of implementation, Ella unplugged the monitor cord from the back of the computer, placed the tablet computer on the desk by the computer, and sat next to Scotty when he sat down by the computer and tried to use it.

Modeling AAC Use and Verbalizations

Modeling of AAC use may serve to provide children with ASD with rich and varied demonstrations of the use of AAC (Binger and Light 2007). AAC instruction that focuses on teaching AAC as output only, such as the Picture Exchange Communication System (Frost and Bondy 2002), tend to rely on spoken language as the only model, failing to provide children with ASD with the multitude of opportunities for language modeling in AAC use, the mode by which they are expected to communicate (Harris and Reichle 2004). This approach, teaching expressive AAC use only, is quite different from the language learning experiences of typically developing children, who continually hear and see others using the modes of verbal (i.e., speech) and nonverbal communication (e.g., facial expressions, tone of voice) they are expected to use (Binger and Light 2007). Unlike output-based AAC interventions, modeling strategies involve modeling of language used via speech and AAC, concomitantly (Drager et al. 2006). The focus of modeling-based interventions is typically primarily on increasing the child's understanding through use of AAC modeling; increased child output via AAC is a desirable side effect (Dada and Alant 2009; Goossens' 1989). Modeling typically involves a facilitator, often an adult, speaking while simultaneously selecting symbols on the person's AAC device (Binger and Light 2007). For example, at dinner time, when the child is eating carrots, the parent might say, "you are eating carrots," while touching to the symbols for

EAT and CARROT. Modeling may occur at the beginning of an activity, following a client's communicative turn, or in an attempt to describe a client's actions (Binger and Light 2007). Efforts should be made to model all of the targeted vocabulary for a given activity (Drager et al. 2006). For example, during play activities, following a child's play action, the adult would select one or more symbols on the child's AAC device, label the symbols at the same time, and then verbally expand on the phrase or words selected (Binger and Light 2007; Mirenda 2008). For example, if the child put a cowgirl figure on a horse, the adult might touch the pictures for *COWGIRL* and *HORSE*, while naming those symbols, and then provide an expanded verbal model ("the cowgirl is riding the horse").

Scenario

When Scotty moved the mouse to try to get the computer to function, Ella selected the HELP symbol on the app and said, "I need help with the computer." Scotty leaned over and peered at the app, but did not touch it.

Expanding, Scaffolding, and Building on Previously Acquired Skills

Naturalistic AAC instruction typically involves following the lead of the person with CCN. Similar to the approach Hart and Risley (1992) noted in parents of typically developing children, language development may be more rapid when communicative partners provide frequent examples of language use by starting with what motivates the children and their current language levels and building on what they already can do. In essence, this involves following children's communicative attempts and expanding on their use of verbal, nonverbal, or AAC-based communications (Binger and Light 2007; Drager et al. 2006). Communication partners may speak in shortened phrases, speak more slowly, provide pauses to allow children to respond, focus on nonverbal communication given by the child, and model expansion of what the children say (Goossens' 1989).

Expanding on the children's communicative attempts may include the following six subcomponents, drawn from the incidental teaching literature (Hart and Risley 1978, 1992). One, communicative partners stay in close proximity with and participate in the activities in which the person is motivated to engage (Hart and Risley 1992). Two, new words and concepts are modeled (Hart and Risley 1992). Specifically, new vocabulary for each activity is planned in advance and icons or words are incorporated into the AAC system, so symbols are ready for use. These new concepts are modeled, as described above, both verbally and via the AAC system. Three, communicative partners repeat what the children communicate, then provide an expansion on what he or she said, such as by adding a descriptor, labeling an item the child did not name correctly, modeling a slightly longer sentence than the child used, using parts of speech not yet acquired by the individual, and incorporating preschool or school curricular content, as appropriate (Speidel and Nelson 1989). Four, attention should be paid to all of the potential communicative functions that a child might need to use in daily interactions (Hart and Risley 1992). These include requesting, commenting and labeling, asking questions for information, responding to questions for information, refusing, requesting assistance, and taking turns in conversation (Wetherby and Prutting 1984). Depending on the functioning level of the individual and given that deficits common in ASD are highly social, socially based communicative functions, such as conversation, may be particularly difficult to teach as they may be less motivating (Baker et al. 1998); thus, it may be necessary to build in other types of motivation, such as having initial conversations around areas of particular interest. Lund and Light (2007) recommend a broad approach, teaching multiple communicative functions simultaneously, unlike some AAC protocols that begin with solely requesting instruction (Frost and Bondy 2002). Five, communicative partners may ask questions related to objects and activities in the immediate environment and to encourage turn-taking in conversation (Hart and Risley 1992). Six, redirection may be useful if the individual is engaging in self-stimulatory behaviors or otherwise not responding to attempts to engage him or her in the activity (Hart and Risley 1992). Above, the importance of motivation to engage in the activity was stressed. If the individual appears to have lost interest, it is up to the communicative partner to find a means to motivate the person to reengage, by changing materials to ones that are more reinforcing or by changing activities, or by ending the communicative exchange on a positive, by providing necessary prompts (see below) or providing a stimulus for a well-mastered skill, to end the interaction on a reinforcing note.

In summary, there are several key components that should be attended to in advance, when planning opportunities for expansion of AAC language skills. New vocabulary that may be needed should be preplanned and programmed into the AAC system. This may relate to activities throughout the daily schedule. For example, there may be the need to request more toothpaste during morning routines if the toothpaste runs out. New communicative functions or functions not applied yet to particular contexts should be considered and pertinent vocabulary added. Advanced language skills that the individual has not mastered, such as parts of speech, should be considered. Finally, if the individual attends school, relevant curricular content must be considered, including any individual goals and objectives, as well as age- or grade-appropriate state or national educational standards.

Implementation of Behavioral Techniques

Behavioral techniques, gleaned from the field of applied behavior analysis, involve direct, strategic teaching of skills, which is necessary when working with individuals with ASD, and those with other DDs, who are less likely to learn from observation than their peers or who may learn more slowly (MacDuff et al. 2001).

Thus, a number of researchers who have implemented naturalistic aided AAC teaching techniques have incorporated behavioral strategies. These techniques include prompts, reinforcement, time delay, and errorless learning.

Prompts are frequently used to teach behaviors that are not currently displayed by the individual with DD or are used infrequently (Akmanoglu and Batu 2004). McMillian (2008) provided physical prompts to students who selected wrong symbols or did not respond to models of AAC use by guiding the student's hand to the correct symbol. Prompts should be faded as soon as possible to avoid prompt dependence (MacDuff et al. 2001), or individuals fail to demonstrate skills independently because prompts are delivered too soon. One way to fade the use of prompts is by increasing the length of the delay using time delay (discussed below). For example, Durand (1999) used physical prompts to teach requesting help and then faded those prompts by waiting 3–5 s for the student to respond. Prompts may be faded by gradually using a less invasive prompt (Binger et al. 2008; MacDuff et al. 2001). Full physical hand-over-hand prompts may be used in initial stages of instruction, such as by helping the individual point and move his hand to the symbol, followed by less intense prompts, such as leading by the wrist, then by the elbow, then with a light tap on the elbow, then no prompt (Cooper 1987). Prompts may also be provided in a least-to-most invasive sequence, such as starting with a verbal prompt (e.g., "tap the FORK picture"), followed by a gestural prompt (e.g., pointing to the FORK picture without selecting it), followed by a physical prompt if the individual does not respond to a less invasive prompt (Johnston et al. 2003).

Reinforcement involves providing a consequence to a behavior that encourages the individual to continue engaging in the behavior or increase the rate of engaging in the behavior (Skinner 1951). In terms of teaching AAC use, a natural positive reinforcer may be handing the person a toy after he or she made a request by selecting a symbol on the AAC device (Cosbey and Johnston 2006). Another example of reinforcement is removing a difficult task when the person selects the I-NEED-A-BREAK symbols. During naturalistic interventions, reinforcement should be provided that is natural for that context or environment, such as attention from peers as a result of using AAC to ask a question or ask to play (Johnston et al. 2003).

Time delay provides the person with ASD with time to respond following the presentation of a stimulus (Reichle et al. 2002; for example, "what state is that?" asked while pointing to Texas on a map, waiting 3 s, then prompting the person to select the symbol for TEXAS). Time delay is frequently used when the individual has the behavior, in this case AAC use, in his or her repertoire, but does not display it frequently or at the correct time. Time delay may be paired with waiting with an expectant look, such as when a communicative temptation has been set up, but the person has not yet initiated an interaction. For example, McMillian (2008) taught teachers to wait 3–10 s for a response when communication opportunities were presented. If the student did not respond or did not respond correctly, the teacher looked expectantly, followed by modeling and prompting as needed. The amount of time must be individualized, based on the person's response latency, or time between a stimulus and a response.

Errorless learning consists of immediately providing necessary prompts to assist the person in a correct response, while preventing incorrect responses (Fillingham et al. 2003). Errorless learning may be used in tandem with time delay; that is, prompts may initially be provided on a 0-s delay (Cosbey and Johnston 2006), gradually increasing the time delay to provide the person with time to respond independently. This technique may be used when teaching initial AAC use by following a stimulus with an immediate prompt (Reichle et al. 2002). For example, to teach someone to select the HELP symbol, Reichle et al. (2002) presented preferred items that the participant could not access and immediately provided physical prompts, guiding the participant's hand to the HELP symbol.

Scenario

Ella waited 5 s after selecting the HELP button, but Scotty did not respond to her model. She then gently took his hand, formed a point, and prompted him to select the HELP symbol. Then, she said, "oh, you need help," while quickly plugging the monitor back in. After he played on the computer for a few minutes, Ella put her clipboard over the screen and asked, "what's that?" while selecting the corresponding symbol on the app and then pointing to the computer. She waited 5 s and then physically prompted Scotty to select the COMPUTER symbol, said, "yes, that's the computer," and moved her clipboard out of the way.

Research Support for Naturalistic Interventions Involving Implementation of Aided AAC with Individuals with ASD and Other DD

Unfortunately, much of the research on the use of naturalistic instructional practices to teach AAC use has been conducted with people who have DD other than ASD. However, it is possible to extrapolate these results, particularly given the common issues people with ASD have with stimulus overselectivity (Cook et al. 1982; Groden and Mann 1988; Huguenin and Touchette 1980), thus providing an impetus for carefully planning implementation of AAC use in numerous contexts versus targeting primarily contrived contexts for intervention. Below, the research on naturalistic instruction in AAC use is described. The first section reviews only studies that included individuals with ASD; however, because of the paucity of research in this area with people with ASD, the following sections include individuals with other DDs and physical impairments as well. Although studies involving the use of implementation in natural contexts and expansion are not explicitly reviewed below, all of the studies involved implementation in natural contexts, providing some instruction on AAC skills the participants did not previously possess, expanding their repertoires. This information is provided so readers have an idea of the literature base for the concepts covered and suggested in this chapter. The studies reviewed in this section are included in Table 5.1.

Table 5.1 Sample of research involving naturalistic aided AAC interventions with people with ASD, DD, and physical impairments

Author(s) (year)	N	Age range (years)	Diagnoses[a]	Participants reported to have some speech[a]	SGD mode(s)[b]	Study design[c]	Setting	Intervention summary	Maintenance or generalization assessed	Results summary
Beck et al. (2009)	6	25–50	DD	Y	PE	SCD-F	Community-based workshop	Modeling aided AAC, music-based intervention	Y	Varied across participants, responsiveness and use of AAC increased
Binger and Light (2007)	5	3–4	OTH, DD	Y	PE	SCD-F	Classroom (n = 3); home (n = 2)	Modeling aided AAC	Y	Four of the five participants learned to consistently produce multi-symbol messages; the fifth did not demonstrate consistent gains
Bruno and Trembath (2006)	9	4–14	OTH	N	PE, SGD-DD	CS/DS	Camp program	Modeling, aided language stimulation	N	Increased syntactic performance when the participants used a manual communication board
Cafiero (2001)	1	13	AU	Y	PE	SCD-F	Middle school SPED classroom/general education school and community	Implementation in natural contexts/activities, natural aided language approach, intense visual-paired-with verbal language input/modeling	N	Increased use of picture language receptive and expressive vocabulary and positive behaviors
Cosbey and Johnston (2006)	3	3.6–6.6	OTH	Y	SGD-SO	SCD	Inclusive classroom setting	Behavioral strategies (prompts, errorless learning, natural reinforcement), implementation in natural contexts/activities	Y	Increased use of SGD to request access to items and peers
Dada and Alant (2009)	4	8.1–12.1	OTH	Y	SGD-DD	SCD	A small room in school for students with ID	Aided language stimulation, implementation in natural contexts/activities	N	Varied results but acquired target vocabulary items

Study	N	Age	Diagnosis		SGD	Design	Setting	Intervention		Outcomes
Dicarlo and Banajee (2000)	2	2–2.6	DD	Y	SGD-SO	SCD-F	Inclusive classroom	Behavioral strategies (prompts), modeling, implementation in natural contexts/activities	N	Increased initiations and unclear initiations and adult prompted communication decreased when the SGDs were used
Drager et al. (2006)	2	4–4.5	AU	Y	PE	SCD	Day care center	Aided language modeling, implementation in natural contexts/activities	Y	Increased symbol comprehension and elicited symbol production and maintained these skills. Performance on symbol production lagged behind symbol comprehension
Durand (1999)	5	3.5–15	AU, MR, OTH	Y	SGD-SO	SCD	SPED classrooms	Behavioral strategies (prompts and graduated guidance), implementation in natural contexts/activities	N	Increased use of SGD while decreasing CB across settings
Dyches (1998)	4	10.4–12.10	AU, ID	Y	SGD-DD	SCD-F	Self-contained classroom	Behavioral strategies (prompts), implementation in natural contexts/activities (coincidental instruction)	N	Increased spontaneous communicative interactions and number of verbalizations
Gordon et al. (2011)	84	4–10	ID, AU	Y	PE	CS	Classroom (snack time)	Implementation in natural contexts/activities, followed PECS training protocol	N	Increased spontaneous communication using picture cards, speech, or both to request objects following training. Spontaneous requesting for social purposes did not increase

(continued)

Table 5.1 (continued)

Author(s) (year)	N	Age range (years)	Diagnoses[a]	Participants reported to have some speech[a]	SGD mode(s)[a]	Study design[b][c]	Setting	Intervention summary	Maintenance or generalization assessed	Results summary
Hamilton and Snell (1993)	1	15	AU, ID	Y	PE	SCD	Classroom, cafeteria, community (mall, grocery store, video arcade, library, restaurant), home	Behavioral strategies (prompts, prompt-fading), modeling, implementation in natural contexts/activities, milieu teaching	Y	Increased use of communication book across settings
Harris and Reichle (2004)	3	3.10–5.4	OTH, no specified diagnosis	Y	PE	SCD	School, home, day care	Behavior strategies (prompt), modeling	Y	Increased symbol comprehension and production
Johnston et al. (2003)	3	4–5	AU, ID, PDD, OTH	Y	PE	SCD	Preschool classroom for children with ASD	Behavioral strategies (prompts, prompt-fading, reinforcement), modeling	Y	Increased prompted and unprompted use of picture symbols
Light et al. (1999)	6	10–44	ID, OTH	Y	SGD-DD	SCD	Sheltered workshop, group home, community settings, disability advocacy group, school, dance class	Behavioral strategies (prompts), modeling, implementation in natural contexts/activities	Y	Increased in asking partner-focused questions spontaneously in social interactions
McMillian (2008)	4	8–12	ID, AU	Y	SGD-DD	SCD-F	SPED classroom	Behavioral strategies (prompts and time delay)	Y	Increased initiations of use of SGD. There was a minimal change in device responses
Ogletree et al. (2012)	1	7	AU	Y	PE	SCD-F	Treatment room in a university speech clinic	Behavioral strategies (prompts), modeling	Y	Increased unprompted photograph exchange

Study	N	Age	Diagnosis		Communication system	Design	Setting	Intervention		Outcomes
Reichle et al. (2002)	1	32	DD	Y	PE	SCD	Group home	Behavioral strategies (time delay, prompts, and errorless learning)	N	Generalizing to other tasks associated escape, but not generalizing to tasks that the learner engaged in CB to obtain preferred but difficult-to-access items
Rodi and Hughes (2000)	1	17	ID, OTH	Y	PE	SCD	Special education classroom, hospital, grocery store	Behavioral strategies (prompts), implementation in natural contexts/ activities, milieu teaching	Y	Increased use of communication book in two settings and more delayed increases in a third setting
Schepis et al. (1998)	4	3, 5	AU	Y	SGD-DD	SCD-F	Self-contained classroom	Behavioral strategies (prompts), modeling	N	Increased communicative interactions using SGD across settings and behaviors
Schepis et al. (1996)	3	23–42	ID, OTH	N	SGD-DD	SCD-F	Training room within adult education program	Behavioral strategies (graduated guidance and time delay)	Y	Increased use of SGD in response to a trainer's request across settings

[a]AU autism, autistic disorder, early infantile autism, DD developmental delay, developmental disorder, ID intellectual disability, mental retardation, PDD/HFA pervasive developmental disorder, not otherwise specified, Asperger syndrome, high functioning autism, "autism spectrum disorder" without a specific diagnosis, SD sensory disability, OTH other disabilities (e.g., chromosomal abnormalities); diagnosis definitions listed here reflect the terms used in the original articles, though they may be outdated

[b]MS manual sign language, PE picture-exchange system (including the Picture Exchange Communication System), SGD-SO speech-generating device or voice output communication aid with single-switch or changeable overlays, SGD-DD speech-generating device or voice output communication aid with dynamic displays, such as computer screens

[c]CS/DS case study, narrative description, or group study with descriptive statistics only, GS group study, SCD single-case design, SCD-F single-case design with significant design flaws

Research with People with ASD

Ten articles were found that included participants in naturalistic AAC interventions; all of these studies included small numbers of participants. The participants in successful studies ranged in age from 3 years (Schepis et al. 1998) to 15 years (Hamilton and Snell 1993), though most involved preschoolers and early elementary-aged children. Unlike many of the studies involving people who did not have ASD that focused primarily on modeling of AAC and verbal skills, most of the studies involving people with ASD included behavioral techniques (Dyches 1998; McMillian 2008), usually in concert with modeling (Johnston et al. 2003; Ogletree et al. 2012; Schepis et al. 1998). There are a small number of studies that involved primarily modeling of AAC use in concert with verbal models, resulting in improvement in expressive and receptive, or comprehension of, communication (Drager et al. 2006). There is a reasonable base of literature to support the implementation of naturalistic strategies with individuals with ASD, particularly when they include behavioral techniques, though there is room for additional research in this area, particularly with adolescents and adults with ASD.

Research Involving Modeling of AAC

At least half of the studies involving naturalistic aided AAC teaching included modeling of AAC use; several of these studies included children with ASD (Cafiero 2001; Drager et al. 2006; Hamilton and Snell 1993; Johnston et al. 2003; Ogletree et al. 2012; Schepis et al. 1998) and most paired modeling with behavioral techniques (Light et al. 1999; Schepis et al. 1998). Many of the studies included verbal modeling paired with AAC modeling (Cafiero 2001; Dada and Alant 2009). Studies were conducted in various natural settings, including craft activities at camp (Bruno and Trembath 2006), cooking (Dada and Alant 2009), play activities (Drager et al. 2006), and conversation (Beck et al. 2009); however, many of the studies limited intervention and data collection to one or two contexts and some did not assess generalization to untrained settings or contexts; thus, results are not easy to generalize to a broad implementation of modeling techniques throughout individuals' daily schedules. Modeling interventions included a wide age range, including adults (Beck et al. 2009), although none of the adults in these studies had ASD and few adults overall were included. Studies primarily included participants who were elementary aged or younger and most were preschool aged (Binger and Light 2007). Overall, studies that included modeling as a component reported success in teaching participants to use, and in some cases to understand, AAC systems.

Research Involving Behavioral Techniques

Many studies involved the use of behavioral techniques. The strategies used in these studies included prompts (Cosbey and Johnston 2006; Light et al. 1999; McMillian 2008). For example, Reichle et al. (2002) taught an adult with severe DD to request help with difficult tasks and to access difficult to access preferred items, using most-to-least intrusive prompts for pointing to a picture. Time delay has also been used in several studies as a means to fade prompts and encourage participants to initiate interactions (McMillian 2008; Ogletree et al. 2012; Reichle et al. 2002; Schepis et al. 1996). Light et al. (1999) taught six individuals with CCN, none of who had ASD, aged 10 to 44 years, to use partner-focused questions that were programmed into their SGDs. Time delay and point prompts were among the behavioral techniques used to teach the participants to use their SGDs. Errorless learning was used in early instructional stages to promote correct responding before prompts were faded (Cosbey and Johnston 2006). Cosbey and Johnston (2006) implemented errorless learning, as well as time delay, prompting, and natural reinforcement, to teach children with severe and multiple disabilities to use SGDs during free-choice activities in inclusive preschool and kindergarten classes.

Conclusions and Future Directions

Scenario

Over the next few weeks, Ella worked with Scotty on labeling a variety of preferred items and asking for help, quickly fading prompts whenever possible. As soon as Scotty demonstrated independent labeling and asking for help for new items, Ella worked with his parents and older brother, assisting them in interacting with Scotty using the app. As he mastered the vocabulary in a variety of settings and with various family members, Ella continued to add new vocabulary and communication functions, including making requests, answering personal questions, and adding descriptors (e.g., color, shape, number of items requested or labeled) and began to work with his parents to determine vocabulary and communication skills needed in the community.

Although there is a need for more research on using naturalistic teaching strategies to teach people with ASD to use AAC, the current base points to several key components that make such strategies well suited for this population, particularly to address the need to ensure individuals with ASD generalize their use of AAC across contexts and communicative functions. It is apparent that the combination of implementation in natural settings, modeling of AAC skills, expansion of current skills, and behavioral techniques would be a powerful approach to meeting their needs. Currently, while no protocol or program exists that explicitly combines these components, caregivers and practitioners who are interested may benefit from instruction in applied behavior analysis, incidental teaching, and using AAC. Some online resources for people interested in these topics are provided in the text box.

Text Box: Resources for Parents and Practitioners

AAC at Penn State: aac.psu.edu
AIM: Autism Internet Modules: www.autisminternetmodules.org

> Applied behavior analysis—an overview
> Incidental teaching
> Naturalistic intervention
> Naturalistic language strategies
> Prompting
> Reinforcement
> Speech-generating devices (SGD)
> Time delay

National Autism Center: www.nationalautismcenter.org
National Professional Development Center on ASD: autismpdc.fpg.unc.edu

Although much progress has been made researching this area, there remains work to be done. In particular, few studies on naturalistic instruction involving aided AAC have included people with ASD (Ganz et al. in press). Further, those that have included individuals with ASD have primarily focused on teaching requesting, rather than a range of communicative functions. Although people with ASD tend to have less interest in purely social interactions than their peers (Lord 1995), research should focus on how to teach the broadest range of communicative functions possible. Naturalistic instruction in AAC, for people with and without ASD, has primarily taken place during play-based activities or meals, limiting their generalizability to other contexts. Finally, a training protocol to assist family members and practitioners in implementing naturalistic AAC instruction should be developed and tested.

References

Akmanoglu, N., & Batu, S. (2004). Teaching pointing to numerals to individuals with autism using simultaneous prompting. *Education and Training in Developmental Disabilities, 39,* 326–336.

Baker, M. J., Koegel, R. L., & Koegel, L. K. (1998). Increasing the social behavior of young children with autism using their obsessive behaviors. *Research and Practice for Persons with Severe Disabilities, 23,* 300–308. doi:10.2511/rpsd.23.4.300.

Beck, A. R., Stoner, J. B., & Dennis, M. L. (2009). An investigation of aided language stimulation: Does it increase AAC use with adults with developmental disabilities and complex communication needs? *Augmentative and Alternative Communication, 25,* 42–54. doi:10.1080/07434610802131059.

Binger, C., Kent-Walsh, J., Berens, J., Del Campo, S., & Rivera, D. (2008). Teaching Latino parents to support the multi-symbol message productions of their children who require AAC. *Augmentative and Alternative Communication, 24,* 323–338. doi:10.1080/07434610802130978.

Binger, C., & Light, J. (2007). The effect of aided AAC modeling on the expression of multi-symbol messages by preschoolers who use AAC. *Augmentative and Alternative Communication, 23*, 30–43. doi:10.1080/07434610600807470.

Bruno, J., & Trembath, D. (2006). Use of aided language stimulation to improve syntactic performance during a weeklong intervention program. *Augmentative and Alternative Communication, 22*, 300–313. doi:10.1080/07434610600768318.

Cafiero, J. M. (2001). The effect of an augmentative communication intervention on the communication, behavior, and academic program of an adolescent with autism. *Focus on Autism and Other Developmental Disabilities, 16*, 179–189. doi:10.1177/108835760101600306.

Calculator, S. N. (1999). AAC outcomes for children and youths with severe disabilities: When seeing is believing. *Augmentative and Alternative Communication, 15*, 4–12. doi:10.1080/074 34619912331278525.

Campbell, J. M. (2003). Efficacy of behavioral interventions for reducing problem behavior in persons with autism: A quantitative synthesis of single-subject research. *Research in Developmental Disabilities, 24*, 120–138. doi:10.1016/S0891-4222(03)00014-3.

Charlop-Christy, M., & Carpenter, M. H. (2000). Modified incidental teaching sessions: A procedure for parents to increase spontaneous speech in their children with autism. *Journal of Positive Behavior Interventions, 2*, 98–112. doi:10.1177/109830070000200203.

Cook, A. R., Anderson, N., & Rincover, A. (1982). Stimulus over-selectivity and stimulus control: Problems and strategies. In R. L. Koegel, A. Rin-cover, & A. L. Egel (Eds.), *Educating and understanding autistic children* (pp. 90–105). San Diego: College-Hill.

Cooper, J. O. (1987). Stimulus control. In J. O. Cooper, T. E. Heron, & W. L. Heward (Eds.), *Applied behavior analysis* (pp. 299–326). Columbus, OH: Merrill.

Cosbey, J. E., & Johnston, S. (2006). Using a single-switch voice output communication aid to increase social access for children with severe disabilities in inclusive classrooms. *Research & Practice for Persons with Severe Disabilities, 31*, 144–156.

Dada, S., & Alant, E. (2009). The effect of aided language stimulation on vocabulary acquisition in children with little or no functional speech. *American Journal of Speech-Language Pathology, 18*, 50–64. doi:10.1044/1058-0360(2008/07-0018).

Dicarlo, C. F., & Banajee, M. (2000). Using voice output devices to increase initiations of young children with disabilities. *Journal of Early Intervention, 23*, 191–199. doi:10.1177/105381510 00230030801.

Drager, K. D. R., Postal, V. J., Carrolus, L., Castellano, M., Gagliano, C., & Glynn, J. (2006). The effect of aided language modeling on symbol comprehension and production in 2 preschoolers with autism. *American Journal of Speech-Language Pathology, 15*, 112–125. doi:10.1044/1058-0360(2006/012).

Durand, V. M. (1999). Functional communication training using assistive devices: Recruiting natural communities of reinforcement. *Journal of Applied Behavior Analysis, 32*, 247–267. doi:10.1901/jaba.1999.32-247.

Dyches, T. T. (1998). Effects of switch training on the communication of children with autism and severe disabilities. *Focus on Autism and Other Developmental Disabilities, 13*, 151–162. doi:10.1177/108835769801300303.

Eldevik, S., Hastings, R. P., Hughes, J. C., Jahr, E., Eikeseth, S., & Cross, S. (2009). Meta-analysis of early intensive behavioral intervention for children with autism. *Journal of Clinical Child and Adolescent Psychology, 38*, 439–450. doi:10.1080/15374410902851739.

Fillingham, J. K., Hodgson, C., Sage, K., & Ralph, M. A. (2003). The application of errorless learning to aphasic disorders: A review of theory and practice. *Neuropsychological Rehabilitation, 13*, 337–363. doi:10.1080/09602010343000020.

Frost, L., & Bondy, A. (2002). *The Picture Exchange Communication System training manual*. Newark, DE: Pyramid Educational Products Incorporated.

Ganz, J. B., Rispoli, M. J., Mason, R. A., & Hong, E. R. (in press). Moderation of effects of AAC based on setting and types of aided AAC on outcome variables: An aggregate study of single-case research with individuals with ASD. *Developmental Neurorehabilitation*. doi: 10.3109/17518423.2012.748097.

Goossens', C. (1989). Aided communication intervention before assessment: A case study of a child with cerebral palsy. *Augmentative and Alternative Communication, 5*, 14–26. doi:10.108 0/07434618912331274926.

Gordon, K., Pasco, G., McElduff, F., Wade, A., Howlin, P., & Charman, T. (2011). A communication-based intervention for nonverbal children with autism: What changes? Who benefits? *Journal of Consulting and Clinical Psychology, 79*, 447–457.

Groden, G., & Mann, L. (1988). Intellectual functioning and assessment. In G. Groden & M. G. Baron (Eds.), *Autism: Strategies for change* (pp. 81–82). New York: Gardner.

Hamilton, B., & Snell, M. (1993). Using the milieu approach to increase spontaneous communication book use across environments by an adolescent with autism. *Augmentative and Alternative Communication, 9*, 259–272. doi:10.1080/07434619312331276681.

Harris, M. D., & Reichle, J. (2004). The impact of aided language stimulation on symbol comprehension and production in children with moderate cognitive disabilities. *American Journal of Speech-Language Pathology, 13*, 155–167. doi:10.1044/1058-0360(2004/016).

Hart, B., & Risley, T. R. (1978). Promoting productive language through incidental teaching. *Education and Urban Society, 10*, 407–429. doi:10.1177/001312457801000402.

Hart, B., & Risley, T. R. (1980). In vivo language intervention: Unanticipated general effects. *Journal of Applied Behavior Analysis, 13*, 407–432. doi:10.1901/jaba.1980.13-407.

Hart, B., & Risley, T. R. (1989). The longitudinal study of interactive systems. *Education and Treatment of Children, 12*, 347–358.

Hart, B., & Risley, T. R. (1992). American parenting of language-learning children: Persisting differences in family-child interactions observed in natural home environments. *Developmental Psychology, 28*, 1096–1105. doi:10.1037/0012-1649.28.6.1096.

Hart, B., & Risley, T. R. (2003). The early catastrophe. The 30 million word gap. *American Educator, 27*, 4–9.

Howlin, P., Magiati, I., & Charman, T. (2009). Systematic review of early intensive behavioral interventions for children with autism. *American Association on Intellectual and Developmental Disabilities, 114*, 23–41. doi:10.1352/2009.114:23-41.

Huguenin, N. H., & Touchette, P. E. (1980). Visual attention in retarded adults: Combining stimuli which control incompatible behavior. *Journal of the Experimental Analysis of Behavior, 33*, 77–86. doi:10.1901/jeab.1980.33-77.

Johnston, S., Nelson, C., Evans, J., & Palazolo, K. (2003). The use of visual supports in teaching young children with autism spectrum disorder to initiate interactions. *Augmentative and Alternative Communication, 19*, 86–103. doi:10.1080/0743461031000112016.

Jonsson, A., Kristoffersson, L., Ferm, U., & Thunberg, G. (2011). The ComAlong communication boards: Parents' use and experiences of aided language stimulation. *Augmentative and Alternative Communication, 27*, 103–116. doi:10.3109/07434618.2011.580780.

King, A. M., & Fahsl, A. J. (2012). Supporting social competence in children who use augmentative and alternative communication. *Teaching Exceptional Children, 45*, 42–49.

Light, J. (1997). "Let's go star fishing": Reflections on the contexts of language learning for children who use aided AAC. *Augmentative and Alternative Communication, 13*, 158–171. doi:10.1080/07434619712331277978.

Light, J. C., Binger, C., Agate, T. L., & Ramsay, K. N. (1999). Teaching partner-focused questions to individuals who use augmentative and alternative communication to enhance their communicative competence. *Journal of Speech, Language, and Hearing Research, 42*, 241–255.

Lord, C. (1995). Follow-up of two-year-olds referred for possible autism. *Journal of Child Psychology and Psychiatry, 36*, 1365–1382. doi:10.1111/j.1469-7610.1995.tb01669.x.

Lund, S. K., & Light, J. (2007). Long-term outcomes for individuals who use augmentative and alternative communication: Part II-communicative interaction. *Augmentative and Alternative Communication, 23*, 1–15. doi:10.1080/07434610600720442.

MacDuff, G. S., Krantz, P. J., & McClannahan, L. E. (2001). Prompts and prompt-fading strategies for people with autism. In C. Maurice, G. Green, & R. M. Foxx (Eds.), *Making a difference: Behavioral intervention for autism*, 37–50. Austin, TX: Pro-Ed., Inc.

McGee, G. G., & Daly, T. (2007). Incidental teaching of age-appropriate social phrases to children with autism. *Research and Practice for Persons with Severe Disabilities, 32*, 112–123. doi:10.2511/rpsd.32.2.112.

McGee, G. G., Morrier, M. J., & Daly, T. (1999). An incidental teaching approach to early intervention for toddlers with autism. *Journal of the Association for Persons with Severe Handicaps, 24*, 133–146. doi:10.2511/rpsd.24.3.133.

McMillian, J. M. (2008). Teachers make it happen: From professional development to integration of augmentative and alternative communication technologies in the classroom. *Australasian Journal of Special Education, 32*, 199–211.

Miranda-Linne, F., & Melin, L. (1992). Acquisition, generalization, and spontaneous use of color adjectives: A comparison of incidental teaching and traditional discrete-trial procedures for children with autism. *Research in Developmental Disabilities, 13*, 191–210. doi:10.1016/0891-4222(92)90025-2.

Mirenda, P. (2008). A back door approach to autism and AAC. *Augmentative and Alternative Commutation, 24*, 220–234.

Mundy, P., Sigman, M., Ungerer, J., & Sherman, T. (1986). Defining the social deficits of autism: The contribution of non-verbal communication measures. *Journal of Child Psychology and Psychiatry, 27*, 657–669. doi:10.1111/j.1469-7610.1986.tb00190.x.

Ogletree, B. T., Davis, P., Hambrecht, G., & Phillips, E. W. (2012). Using milieu training to promote photograph exchange for a young child with autism. *Focus on Autism and Other Developmental Disabilities, 27*, 93–101. doi:10.1177/1088357612441968.

Reichle, J., Drager, K., & Davis, C. (2002). Using requests for assistance to obtain desired items and to gain release from nonpreferred activities: Implications for assessment and intervention. *Education and Treatment of Children, 25*, 47–66.

Rodi, M. S., & Hughes, C. (2000). Teaching communication book use to a high school student using a milieu approach. *Research and Practice for Persons with Severe Disabilities, 25*, 175–179. doi:10.2511/rpsd.25.3.175.

Romski, M. A., Sevcik, R. A., & Robinson, B. R. (1996). Mapping the meaning of novel visual symbols by youth with moderate or severe mental retardation. *American Journal on Mental Retardation, 100*, 391–402.

Schepis, M. M., Reid, D. H., & Behrman, M. M. (1996). Acquisition and functional use of voice output communication by persons with profound multiple disabilities. *Behavior Modification, 20*, 451–468. doi:10.1177/01454455960204005.

Schepis, M. M., Reid, D. H., Behrmann, M. M., & Sutton, K. A. (1998). Increasing communicative interactions of young children with autism using a voice output communication aid and naturalistic teaching. *Journal of Applied Behavior Analysis, 31*, 561–578. doi:10.1901/jaba.1998.31-561.

Sevcik, R. A., Romski, M. A., & Watkins, R. V. (1995). Adult partner-augmented communication input to youth with mental retardation using the system for augmenting language (SAL). *Journal of Speech and Hearing Research, 38*, 902–912.

Skinner, B. F. (1951). How to teach animals. *Scientific American, 185*, 26–29.

Speidel, G. E., & Nelson, K. E. (Eds.). (1989). *The many faces of imitation in language learning.* Berlin: Springer.

Veness, C., Prior, M., Bavin, E., Eadie, P., Cini, E., & Reilly, S. (2012). Early indicators of autism spectrum disorders at 12 and 24 months of age: A prospective, longitudinal comparative study. *Autism: The International Journal of Research and Practice, 16*, 163–177. doi:10.1177/1362361311399936.

Wetherby, A., & Prutting, C. (1984). Profiles of communicative and cognitive-social abilities in autistic children. *Journal of Speech and Hearing Research, 27*, 364–377.

Chapter 6
AAC Intervention Mediated by Natural Communication Partners

Jennifer B. Ganz and Ee Rea Hong

Introduction

Considering training for natural communication partners, including peers and family members, is critical when implementing AAC with students with CCN (Fisher and Shogren 2012). Further, just as it is critical for students who use AAC to communicate with teachers and parents, communicating with peers is also a critical daily activity (King and Fahsl 2012). Given that social deficits are a key characteristic of ASD (American Psychiatric Association [APA] 2013), and that this population is unlikely to initiate interactions with others or to learn skills incidentally from observing others, it is particularly critical to provide instruction for common natural communication partners to encourage interactions between people with ASD and others. When peers are untrained, the rate of interactions with their classmates with CCN is typically low (Chung and Carter 2013; Fisher and Shogren 2012). Although there is less research involving family members, the same patterns can be assumed to be true comparing interactions between typically developing family members versus those with ASD. Thus, interventions for people with ASD, including those involving AAC, should include family members and peers as key partners. This chapter focuses on interventions that involved parents and peers in AAC interventions, excluding studies with teachers, which are far more common.

> **Scenario**
>
> Chen received a 6-weeks report on the progress of her eighth grade son, Park, who had ASD and CCN. According to the report, Park used a picture exchange-based AAC system at school and had mastered using it to request food at lunch time and magazines and the iPad to use when he completed class work. He also reportedly responded to questions about activities happening at school.

(continued)

(continued)

Although Park brought his communication binder home every day, Chen and Park's stepfather, Ben, had never seen Park take it out of his backpack to use it for anything at home. Chen sent a note to school, asking his teacher, Alexa, if they could schedule a meeting to discuss how to get Park to use the AAC system at home more often. After a brief teacher conference, Alexa suggested they start with six, once-per-week 1 h sessions of parent and home training and said she was available and willing to come to their home to help Park generalize his use of his communication book to his home and with his family. Park's educational team agreed with this suggestion and wrote it into his educational plan.

The Case for Involving Parents, Family Members, and Peers in AAC Intervention

Students with CCN, including those with ASD and ID, far more frequently communicate with support staff in the classroom than with peers (Clarke and Wilkinson 2008), even when proximity to peers is as frequent as proximity to adults; this is very different from the rates of social interactions with peers for typically developing students (Chung et al. 2012). This is particularly striking when considering students with ASD versus others with DD; Chung et al. (2012) found that half of their participants with ASD did not interact with peers during any observations, although nearly all of the students with ID did. It appears that without direct instruction in peer-mediated AAC interventions, interactions between children with ASD and their peers will be limited.

General education teachers who have students who use AAC in their classrooms note a number of barriers to successful inclusion of these students, including lack of training for teachers and instructional assistants in how to implement AAC, a low rate of interactions between students who use AAC and their peers, limitations on the part of the devices, and lack of skills in using AAC devices on the part of students with CCN (Kent-Walsh and Light 2003). Among other issues, it seems apparent that breakdowns in communication may be common between children using AAC and their peers, although typically developing children may learn to manage these issues via asking questions for understanding and prompting the speaker, such as by asking if they mean to say what was communicated via the AAC device (Clarke and Wilkinson 2008).

Peer-mediated strategies are implemented because peers are considered to be ideally situated to assist young people with ASD in practicing social and communication skills in natural settings and because instruction with natural communication partners and in natural settings is the best way to promote generalization of skills across contexts and maintenance of skills over time (Ganz et al. 2008; Sawyer, et al. 2005).

In fact, peer relationships typically develop outside of adult supervision; thus, peers may be the ideal interventionists (Simpson et al. 2012). Further, specific to AAC, typically developing students have been found to have more favorable attitudes toward their peers with CCN when those peers use SGDs (Lilienfeld and Alant 2002).

Parents are considered to be the first, and frequently, the best teachers children have; this is particularly important when a family member has ASD because that individual may require advocacy throughout the lifespan to ensure access to needed services (Hendricks and Wehman 2009). Parent coaching and parent-mediated AAC interventions for people with CCN have reported a number of positive outcomes for family members, including beyond instruction in particular skills. When provided with instruction regarding how to use AAC with their children, including some who had ASD, parents report positive impacts on their children's language development and their abilities to communicate with one another, particularly because the parents modified their speech to provide better, more concise models to their children and modeling of AAC use (Jonsson et al. 2011). Further, parent coaching in SGD interventions is associated with parent perceptions of decreases in severity of their children's language delays and improvements in speech skills among children who use some spoken words spontaneously (Romski et al. 2011; Smith et al. 2011). Parents' perceptions of the severity of their children's communication deficits are also correlated with their parental stress level (Smith et al. 2011); thus, because parent-coached AAC interventions result in perception of less severity, providing parent-mediated AAC intervention may result in decreased parental stress.

Although parent-mediated AAC interventions may have positive outcomes, it is important to consider particular family priorities and needs and provide parents with information on why AAC is recommended (Marshall and Goldbart 2008). Any interventions, including AAC interventions, that appear to the parents to be an added requirement become an added stressor. Further, some parents note that they wish to be respected for their expertise of their children and their children's communication styles and skills and that their choices should be considered when making decisions regarding AAC use (Marshall and Goldbart 2008). Thus, parent-mediated interventions should be preceded with a discussion with family members regarding their priorities and how they would be fit into the context of an AAC intervention.

Description of Peer- and Parent-Mediated AAC Interventions

Simply, interventions that involve natural communication partners include any educational or behavioral interventions that are mediated, or implemented, by the communication partners that individuals with ASD would typically encounter in daily life.

Many of the recommendations below apply to both parent-mediated and peer-mediated interventions; however, while parents are typically experts in their children's communication characteristics, peers typically are not and may require additional information. The following are recommendations for the implementation of peer- and parent-mediated interventions; they should be individualized based on the communication partner(s) prior level of understanding and knowledge. Peer- and parent-mediated interventions should include the following key components: (a) information about ASD and CCN and on AAC, (b) instruction and coaching in the selected intervention to be implemented by the peer or parent, and (c) implementation within natural contexts, the last of which was covered in the previous chapter.

Information About ASD and CCN and on AAC

Peers, and sometimes parents, often need information on ASD and AAC in general and on the specific characteristics of their particular classmate or child and the specific type of AAC used (Beck and Fritz-Verticchio 2003). Information about ASD should be provided in an age-appropriate manner and may be provided in large groups, small groups, or one-on-one (King and Fahsl 2012). For example, kindergarten children may participate in a group discussion of strengths and weaknesses everybody has, including themselves, eventually leading to a discussion of strengths and weakness specific to ASD. High school students may be provided with more technical information regarding the characteristics of ASD, including the range of functioning levels. Any age could benefit from the use of age-appropriate commercial video discussing the characteristics with real-life examples. If parents of individuals with ASD consent, such discussions might include conversations about an individual student in particular and his or her communication needs. Family members themselves may wish to sit on panels or in small group discussions to share stories about how they overcome communication barriers.

Similarly, natural communication partners would benefit from information about what AAC is and the purpose of using AAC (Beck and Fritz-Verticchio 2003; King and Fahsl 2012). In particular, parents should be involved in decisions about the best form of AAC for their children. School personnel may provide information on the range of options and recommendations based on formal and informal assessment results and the evidence base, but the needs of the family should be considered. Specific information should be provided regarding the particular AAC device used by the individual with ASD; the person with ASD and CCN might provide a demonstration of how he or she uses his or her AAC device. Family members and peers can be introduced to the types of symbols used, how the AAC device works, and how the child selects messages (Binger et al. 2008). Further, parents may be involved in programming the device and should be provided with information and resources regarding how to select and organize images or concepts. Finally, it may be beneficial to explain to peers the difficulties that may arise for their classmate who uses AAC and how they may help him or her overcome these barriers (King and Fahsl 2012).

Scenario

During Alexa's first home visit, she asked Chen and Ben what they already knew about the purpose of AAC, how Park's picture system worked, when they felt AAC could be used, what concerns they had about using AAC, what barriers they noted with using AAC in the home, and if they had any questions. She found out that Chen had attended some sessions at a parent conference on autism and at the state professional conference on applied behavior analysis and that she felt she had a basic understanding of what AAC was. Chen had some concerns about AAC. One, she was concerned that carrying around the communication book in public might make Park look different from the other kids. Two, Chen was not sure how they would find time to implement AAC throughout their busy schedule that included one older and one younger son, both of whom had after school activities several days each week. Three, Chen was not sure how to get Park to use his communication book spontaneously. However, she and Ben did want Park to learn to communicate more at home, particularly during meals, related to chores he was expected to do, to make choices during free time, and to make his needs known more appropriately.

Alexa also asked Chen and Ben if there were particular times of day or activities during which Park seemed to get frustrated and communication broke down. Park's parents were both involved in all aspects of parenting their children. Chen was an ER doctor and on days when she was working the early morning shift, Ben got Park ready for school. They noted that they often had difficulties getting Park to dress in weather-appropriate clothing, particularly in the winter. Park would dress himself in shorts, even when the temperature was close to freezing, and run away from Ben or Chen when they tried to offer him warmer clothes. Chen thought the issue was related to routine—Park did not understand that when the weather changed, it meant that he needed to wear long sleeves and pants—and because he found certain textures of clothing to be constraining and uncomfortable.

Because of the varied contexts in which Chen and Ben felt Park's communication needs should be addressed, Alexa suggested a multimodal approach. Park had a tablet computer and Chen had already downloaded an AAC app on it. For example, Alexa suggested that they use that when they were out in the community and needed a flexible means of finding necessary vocabulary on the spot. Related to dressing in the morning, she suggested teaching Park to say no by shaking his head when offered something he did not want, such as an item of clothing or food, and using a clothing choice board to be kept near his closet. The board would include picture-based instructions for winter-appropriate and summer-appropriate clothing along with the universal NO symbol to attach over the wrong clothes for the season. There would be a separate choice board for winter clothing and one for summer clothing and each board would have photos of options for tops and bottoms so Park could select what he wanted to wear. Chen and Ben were on board with these ideas (Fig. 6.1).

(continued)

(continued)

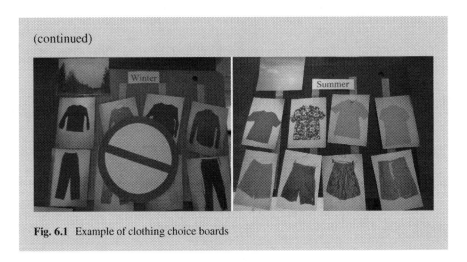

Fig. 6.1 Example of clothing choice boards

Instruction and Coaching in the Intervention

Peer- and parent-mediated strategies for individuals with ASD often entail providing typically developing peers and family members with instructions and practice in implementing interventions with their classmates with ASD (Ganz et al. 2013; Goldstein et al. 2007; Simpson et al. 2012). Interventions that include natural communication partners may include any evidence-based intervention with the addition of training for laypersons. Teaching explicit strategies to encourage communication may be particularly useful in promoting AAC use between peers and people with ASD and CCN (Goldstein et al. 2007). The interventions implemented with the peers or parents will vary depending on their ages and abilities. That is, young peers or siblings, such as those in preschool or early elementary grades (Ganz and Flores 2008), would be expected to implement simple, perhaps single-step, interventions, while adult parents and family members and adolescent peers could be expected to implement slightly more complex interventions, such as those involving many steps or more complex directions (Ganz et al. 2012). Self-monitoring strategies, such as checklists and token boards, may be used to increase independent implementation and reduce the need for teacher or practitioner prompting (Sainato et al. 1992). The specific teaching objectives and interventions implemented will depend on the needs of the target individual. Specific techniques are recommended in Chap. 5.

When peers or parents are introduced to strategies to increase interactions, practitioners should consider the following concepts (Goldstein et al. 2007). One, peers may be introduced to the particular strategies by name and told what they are expected to do. Two, interventionists can give them opportunities to role-play to practice implementing newly taught mediation skills, in this case, AAC-based interactions (Beck and Fritz-Verticchio 2003). The parent or peer should be provided with corrective feedback along with positive reinforcement for correct implementation. Three, because communication skills are typically an area of concern with people with ASD, particularly those with CCN, peers and parents may be taught to prompt and respond to communicative behaviors and to provide other supports (Goldstein et al. 2007). This may include teaching expansions strategies, such as those recommended in Chap. 5, and specific social interaction objectives, such as making and responding to eye contact (Carter and Maxwell 1998; Goldstein and Wickstrom 1986; Light et al. 1992), initiating and responding to joint attention bids (Light et al. 1992), modeling and prompting AAC use (Johnston et al. 2003), asking questions of their peers (Carter and Maxwell 1998; Goldstein and Wickstrom 1986), providing wait time and allowing for slower interaction (Grether and Sickman 2008), joining into the person's preferred activities and play, focusing on responsiveness to the person with CCN instead of giving directions (Light et al. 1992, 1999), asking for clarification or more information to repair communication breakdowns (Grether and Sickman 2008), and commenting on the specific activities and items with which the person with ASD is engaging (Goldstein et al. 1992; Goldstein and Wickstrom 1986).

The following are additional guidelines for increasing the integration of students with CCN in inclusive classrooms. One, plan and initiate cooperative group activities in which all students have a role, establish familiar communication routines that require turn-taking around familiar topics (e.g., board games) (Ratcliff and Cress 1999). Two, ensure that concrete objects are available to support conversational turns related to present activities or conversations (e.g., personal photo albums) (Ratcliff and Cress 1999). Three, encourage classroom dynamics that increase interactions between small groups of students (Ratcliff and Cress 1999).

Scenario

Once the communication boards were in place around their home and the communication app was programmed to include critical vocabulary, Alexa worked with Chen and Ben to assist them in implementing the new techniques. For example, to implement the wardrobe choice board, Alexa came one morning and demonstrated for Chen and Ben how to use it to communicate with Park about his choices. She also brought a checklist listing the steps of using it. It included the following steps:

1. Point to the correct weather icon and tell Park, "It's summer/winter. We have to wear short/long sleeves and shorts/pants"
2. Point to the list of choices of clean tops and tell Park, "Pick one."

   2a. If Park does not make a choice, take his hand and lead it to the options and help him pick one.
   2b. If Park does not make a choice after a physical prompt, take a photo of an item off the chart and ask if he would like that item. If he communicates that he does not want it, model and head shake for "no" and physically prompt him to shake his head. If he takes the picture or otherwise communicates that he wants it, model and physically prompt a "yes" nod.

3. Show Park where that shirt is and help him take it off the hanger.

(continued)

(continued)
4. After Park puts on the top, repeat the procedure for the bottoms.
5. If Park tries to choose the wrong season's clothing, point to the no symbol covering the incorrect season and remind Park, "No shorts/pants today."

She read aloud from the checklist as she went through each step. The following day, Alexa came and asked Ben to implement the steps with her feedback and support. Then, she came the following week to check in.

Research

There is a paucity of research involving peer-mediated interventions for people with IDD and CCN that involve implementation of AAC; among the research in this area, there is a particular dearth of research involving studies that intervene with both the individual with CCN and peers (Fisher and Shogren 2012). Below are summaries of some of the research on peer-mediated interventions for people with ASD, peer- and parent-mediated AAC interventions for people with ASD, and peer- and parent-mediated AAC interventions for people with other disabilities.

Peer-Mediated Interventions for ASD

Peer-mediated interventions to teach socio-communicative skills to individuals with ASD have become accepted and have seen an uptick of support in the research literature (Ganz and Flores 2010a, b; Owen-DeSchryver et al. 2008; Simpson et al. 2012). Research demonstrating the usefulness of peer-mediated interventions for young children with ASD was first reported in the literature in the 1970s (Strain 1977; Strain et al. 1977, 1979). Studies involving peer-mediated strategies in naturalistic contexts have been well studied, particularly for young children with ASD and in comparison to other types of social skill instruction (Matson et al. 2007; Simpson et al. 2012). This assertion is supported by the *National Standards Project* (National Autism Center 2009), which categorized peer training as an established treatment.

To date, peer-mediated interventions have significant support across a number of studies. Unfortunately, much of this research has been limited to implementation with children aged 10 years and younger. For example, recently, Strain and Bovey (2011) reported the results of a randomized controlled trial investigating the LEAP preschool program, which incorporates peer mediation and naturalistic instruction, finding that LEAP participants had better outcomes in severity of autism characteristics, cognitive measures, and language when compared to their peers. One recent study evaluated a peer-mediated visual script intervention with a middle school student and two peers (Ganz et al. 2012). Further, peer-mediated research with people with ASD has investigated limited outcome measures, primarily including play skills (Ganz and Flores 2008; Goldstein et al. 1992), verbal communication (Ganz and Flores 2008; Thiemann and Goldstein 2004), social initiations (Owen-DeSchryver et al. 2008), and sharing (Sawyer et al. 2005). The following interventions or strategies have been taught to or used with peers to increase interaction with their classmates with ASD: models and role playing (Goldstein et al. 1992), prompts for peers to interact (Sawyer et al. 2005), positive reinforcement (Sawyer et al. 2005), visual scripts (Ganz and Flores 2008; Ganz et al. 2012; Thiemann and Goldstein 2004), and other visual supports (Ganz and Flores 2008; Goldstein et al. 1992).

Peer- and Parent-Mediated AAC Interventions for ASD

This review of the literature includes studies in which parents, caregivers, or peers served as interventionists in some way. That is, studies were excluded if educators or researchers taught the participants to use AAC or data were merely collected with parents or peers, but studies in which parents or peers were instructed to use prompts or other strategies to encourage AAC use in the person with ASD were included. Further, studies that involved implementation of parent- or peer-mediated AAC interventions that did not provide measures of child outcomes and/or treatment integrity (i.e., correct implementation of the intervention), such as those measuring parent perceptions of treatment (Romski et al. 2011; Smith et al. 2011), are not included in this review. Table 6.1 provides summaries of studies that investigated the use of parent- or peer-mediated AAC interventions for people with ASD.

We were able to locate some articles that involved implementation of AAC with natural communication partners. Similarly to the broader base of literature on peer-mediated interventions for people with ASD, the studies were primarily implemented with children aged 12 years (Sigafoos et al. 2004) and younger, particularly preschoolers (Nelson et al. 2007; Trembath et al. 2009). Although research is needed with older individuals, it is promising that even young children can successfully support communication of their peers with ASD (Trembath et al. 2009). As might be expected, the AAC-based peer- and parent-mediated interventions primarily involved outcomes relating to communication (Park et al. 2011; Trottier et al. 2011); however, some also reported increases in social engagement (Garrison-Harrell et al. 1997; Thunberg et al. 2009b) and play skills (Nelson et al. 2007). A number of strategies have been implemented to encourage parent and peer mediation of AAC use. Most studies have used some combination of behavioral strategies (see Chap. 5), such as modeling (Nelson et al. 2007), prompts (Ben Chaabane et al. 2009; Nunes and Hanline 2007; Sigafoos et al. 2004), and positive reinforcement (Park et al. 2011), and many involved implementation in natural contexts (Thunberg et al. 2009a, b; Trembath et al. 2009). Interventions research included approximately equal numbers of studies involving peers (Garrison-Harrell et al. 1997; Trottier et al. 2011) and parents (Nunes and Hanline 2007; Thunberg et al. 2009a, b). In some cases, parents reportedly had high rates of treatment integrity (Ben Chaabane et al. 2009).

Table 6.1 Peer- and parent-mediated AAC interventions for ASD

Author(s) (year)	N	Age range (years)	Diagnoses[a]	Participants reported to have some speech	SGD mode(s)[b]	Study design[c]	Intervention summary	Parent or peer-mediated?	Maintenance or generalization assessed	Results summary
Ben Chaabane et al. (2009)	2	5–6	AU	N	PE	SCD	Behavioral strategies (prompting, verbal feedback)	Parent	Y	Increased in correct improvisations during follow-up probes across categories
Garrison-Harrell et al. (1997)	3	6–7	AU	Y	PE	SCD	Peer networks: behavioral strategies (prompting)	Peer	N	Increased social interaction time, use of AAC system, and expressive language
McConkey et al. (2010)	61	2–3	AU	N	PE	G	TEACCH (instructions were given based on PECS protocol)	Parent	N	Increased communication skills Mother participants reported less stress and more satisfaction with their child
Nelson et al. (2007)	4	3–4	AU	Y	PE MS	SCD	Play intervention: behavioral strategies (promoting, modeling) Natural context/activities	Peer	Y	Increased play initiations and engagement time in playgroups
Nunes and Hanline (2007)	1	4	AU	N	PE	SCD-F	Natural context/ activities (environmental arrangement) Behavior strategies (mand/comment with AAC, modeling)	Parent	Y	Increased mother's use of naturalistic strategies Increased communication and use of AAC modes and no change in use of imitative responses
Park et al. (2011)	3	2	AU	Y	PE	SCD-F	Behavioral strategies (PECS protocol: prompt, reinforcement, modeling)	Parent	Y	Increase in independent use of PECS and generalized the skills to different persons, but limited improvement in vocalizations

Study										Outcomes
Sigafoos et al. (2004)	1	12	AU	Y	SGD-DD	SCD-F	Behavioral strategies (verbal feedback, prompt)	Parent	Y	Increased use of AAC mode to make requests across settings
Thunberg et al. (2009a)	4	4–7	AU, PDD/HFA	Y	SGD-DD	SCD-F	Behavioral strategies (modeling, prompt)	Parent	N	Increased the contributions within the topic of the ongoing activity and conversation length between the children participants and their parents; decreased unrelated conversation from the topic
Thunberg et al. (2009b)	3	4–7	AU, PDD/HFA	Y	SGD-DD	SCD-F	Natural context/activities Behavioral strategies (modeling)	Parent	N	Increased in engagement in activity, role taking, and initiations; decreased in use of paralinguistic forms of communication
Trembath et al. (2009)	3	3–5	AU	Y	SGD-DD	SCD	Natural context/ activities Behavioral strategies (modeling, prompt)	Peer	Y	Increased in communicative behaviors and interactions with peers
Trottier et al. (2011)	2	11	AU	Y	SGD-DD	SCD-F	Behavioral strategies (prompt)	Peer	N	Peers were able to acquire skills to support AAC use; increased in use of spontaneous communicative acts

[a] AU autism, autistic disorder, early infantile autism, DD developmental delay, developmental disability, ID intellectual disability, mental retardation, PDD/HFA pervasive developmental disorder, not otherwise specified, Asperger syndrome, high functioning autism, "autism spectrum disorder" without a specific diagnosis, SD sensory disability, OTH other disabilities (e.g., chromosomal abnormalities); diagnosis definitions listed here reflect the terms used in the original articles, though they may be outdated

[b] MS manual sign language, PE picture-exchange system (including the Picture Exchange Communication System), SGD-SO speech-generating device or voice output communication aid with single-switch or changeable overlays, SGD-DD speech-generating device or voice output communication aid with dynamic displays, such as computer screens

[c] CS case study, narrative description, G group study, SCD robust single-case design, SCD-F single-case design with significant design flaws

Peer- and Parent-Mediated AAC Interventions for Anyone with Disabilities

Some research also exists involving implementation of AAC with natural communication partners of individuals with disabilities other than ASD; these included a variety of disabilities, such as cerebral palsy (Carter and Maxwell 1998) and Down syndrome (Kent-Walsh et al. 2010). These studies were implemented with a wide range of age groups, including one with an adult and her mother (Cheslock et al. 2008). The interventions primarily involved outcomes relating to communication (Binger et al. 2008; Cheslock et al. 2008); although some reported improvements in social engagement (Adamson et al. 2010; Carter and Maxwell 1998). The strategies involved behavioral strategies (Chung and Carter 2013; Hunt et al. 1991) and implementation in natural contexts (Kent-Walsh et al. 2010; Lilienfeld and Alant 2005); a couple of studies involved storybook reading (Binger et al. 2008). Interventions included parents (Adamson et al. 2010; Kent-Walsh et al. 2010) more often than peers (Chung and Carter 2013; Lilienfeld and Alant 2005) (Table 6.2).

Conclusions

As noted above, family members and peers are the natural communication partners most often encountered by people with ASD and CNN; thus, it is imperative for them to be involved in interactions via AAC (Ben Chaabane et al. 2009). Because social deficits are a core characteristic in ASD, and these individuals may not frequently initiate interactions, targeted interventions are needed, particularly those that include natural communicative partners as implementers (Ganz et al. 2013; Light 1997). In addition to the above information and that in the previous chapter, the text box provides parents and practitioners with some resources that may be useful in providing instructions and training for implementation of AAC with natural communication partners.

Text Box: Resources for Parents and Practitioners

AAC at Penn State: aac.psu.edu
AIM: Autism Internet Modules: www.autisminternetmodules.org

> Applied behavior analysis—an overview
> Incidental teaching
> Naturalistic intervention
> Naturalistic language strategies
> Prompting
> Reinforcement
> Speech-generating devices (SGD)
> Time delay

National Autism Center: www.nationalautismcenter.org
National Professional Development Center on ASD: autismpdc.fpg.unc.edu

Table 6.2 Peer- and parent-mediated AAC interventions for other disabilities

Author(s) (year)	N	Age range (years)	Diagnoses[a]	Participants reported to have some speech	SGD mode(s)[b]	Study design[c]	Intervention summary	Parent or peer mediated?	Maintenance or generalization assessed	Results summary
Adamson et al. (2010)	57	2–3	DD	N	SGD not specified	G	Communication play protocol not specified	Parent	N	Increased symbol-infused joint engagement
Binger et al. (2008)	3	2–4	OTH	Y	SGD-DD	SCD	Behavioral strategies (modeling, delayed prompt)	Parent	Y	Increased use of strategy and use of symbol combinations
Carter and Maxwell (1998)	4	5–9	OTH	Y	PE	SCD-F	Natural context/activities Behavioral strategies (prompt, reinforcement)	Peer	N	Increased social interactions The peer participants implemented the strategies consistently
Cheslock et al. (2008)	1	30	ID	Y	SGD-DD	CS	Natural context/activities Behavioral strategies (modeling)	Parent	N	Increased communication skills and interactions with others
Chung and Carter (2013)	2	11–12	ID	Y	SGD-DD	SCD	Behavioral strategies (prompt)	Peer	N	Increased the peer interaction across settings
Hunt et al. (1991)	3	15–19	ID, OTH	Y	PE	SCD-F	Behavioral strategies (prompt-fade)	Peer	Y	Increased number of conversational turn-taking and generalized the skills across persons
Kent-Walsh et al. (2010)	6	4–8	OTH	Y	SGD-DD	SCD	Natural context/activities	Parent	Y	The mother participants implemented the strategies with high accuracy Increased number of turn-taking
Lilienfeld and Alant (2005)	1	15	OTH	Y	PE SGD-DD	CS	Behavioral strategies (prompt) Natural context/activities not specified	Peer	Y	Increased social interactions with the peers and the number of messages per interchange

[a] *AU* autism, autistic disorder, early infantile autism, *DD* developmental delay, developmental disability, *ID* intellectual disability, mental retardation, *PDD/HFA* pervasive developmental disorder, not otherwise specified, Asperger syndrome, high functioning autism, "autism spectrum disorder" without a specific diagnosis, *SD* sensory disability, *OTH* other disabilities (e.g., chromosomal abnormalities); diagnosis definitions listed here reflect the terms used in the original articles, though they may be outdated

[b] *MS* manual sign language, *PE* picture-exchange system (including the Picture Exchange Communication System), *SGD-SO* speech-generating device or voice output communication aid with single-switch or changeable overlays, *SGD-DD* speech-generating device or voice output communication aid with dynamic displays, such as computer screens

[c] *CS* case study, narrative description, *G* group study, *SCD* robust single-case design, *SCD-F* single-case design with significant design flaws

References

Adamson, L. B., Romski, M., Bakeman, R., & Sevcik, R. A. (2010). Augmented language intervention and the emergence of symbol-infused joint engagement. *Journal of Speech, Language & Hearing Research, 53*, 1769–1773. doi:10.1044/1092-4388(2010/09-0208).

American Psychiatric Association [APA]. (2013). *Diagnostic and statistical manual* (5th ed.). Washington, DC: Author.

Beck, A. R., & Fritz-Verticchio, H. (2003). The influence of information and role-playing experiences on children's attitudes toward peers who use AAC. *American Journal of Speech-Language Pathology, 12*, 51–58.

Ben Chaabane, D. B., Alber-Morgan, S., & DeBar, R. M. (2009). The effects of parent-implemented PECS training on improvisation of mands by children with autism. *Journal of Applied Behavior Analysis, 42*, 671–677.

Binger, C., Kent-Walsh, J., Berens, J., Del Campo, S., & Rivera, D. (2008). Teaching Latino parents to support the multi-symbol message productions of their children who require AAC. *Augmentative and Alternative Communication, 24*, 323–338. doi:10.1080/07434610802130978.

Carter, M., & Maxwell, K. (1998). Promoting interaction with children using augmentative communication through a peer-directed intervention. *International Journal of Disability, Development & Education, 45*, 75–96. doi:10.1080/1034912980450106.

Cheslock, M. A., Barton-Hulsey, A., Romski, M., & Sevcik, R. A. (2008). Using a speech-generating device to enhance communicative abilities for an adult with moderate intellectual disability. *Intellectual and Developmental Disabilities, 46*, 376–386.

Chung, Y. E., & Carter, E. W. (2013). Promoting peer interactions in inclusive classrooms for students who use speech-generating devices. *Research & Practice for Persons with Severe Disabilities, 38*, 94–109.

Chung, Y., Carter, E. W., & Sisco, L. G. (2012). Social interactions of students with disabilities who use augmentative and alternative communication in inclusive classrooms. *American Journal on Intellectual and Developmental Disabilities, 117*, 349–367.

Clarke, M., & Wilkinson, R. (2008). Interaction between children with cerebral palsy and their peers 2: Understanding initiated VOCA-mediated turns. *Augmentative and Alternative Communication, 24*, 3–15. doi:10.1080/07434610701390400.

Fisher, K. W., & Shogren, K. A. (2012). Integrating augmentative and alternative communication and peer support for students with disabilities: A social-ecological perspective. *Journal of Special Education Technology, 27*, 23–39.

Ganz, J. B., & Flores, M. M. (2008). Effects of the use of visual strategies in play groups for children with autism spectrum disorders and their peers. *Journal of Autism and Developmental Disorders, 38*, 926–940. doi:10.1007/s10803-007-0463-4.

Ganz, J. B., & Flores, M. M. (2010a). Implementing visual cues for young children with autism spectrum disorders and their classmates. *Young Children, 65*, 78–83.

Ganz, J. B., & Flores, M. M. (2010b). Supporting the play of preschoolers with autism spectrum disorders: Implementation of visual scripts. *Young Exceptional Children, 13*, 58–70. doi:10.1177/1096250609351795.

Ganz, J. B., Goodwyn, F. D., Boles, M. B., Hong, E. R., Rispoli, M. J., Lund, E. M., & Kite, E. (2013). Impacts of PECS instructional coaching intervention on practitioners and children with autism. *Augmentative and Alternative Communication, 29*, 210–221. doi:10.3109/07434618.2013.818058.

Ganz, J. B., Heath, A. K., Lund, E. M., Camargo, S., Rispoli, M. J., Boles, M. B., & Plaisance, L. (2012). Effects of peer-mediated visual scripts in middle school. *Behavior Modification, 36*, 378–398. doi:10.1177/0145445512442214.

Ganz, J. B., Sigafoos, J., Simpson, R. L., & Cook, K. E. (2008). Generalization of a pictorial alternative communication system across instructors and distance. *Augmentative and Alternative Communication, 24*, 89–99.

Garrison-Harrell, L., Kamps, D., & Kravits, T. (1997). The effects of peer networks on social-communicative behaviors for students with autism. *Focus on Autism and Other Developmental Disabilities, 12*, 241–254.

Goldstein, H., Kaczmarek, L., Pennington, R., & Shafer, K. (1992). Peer-mediated intervention: Attending to, commenting on, and acknowledging the behavior of preschoolers with autism. *Journal of Applied Behavior Analysis, 25*, 289–305. doi:10.1901/jaba.1992.25-289.

Goldstein, H., Schneider, N., & Thiemann, K. (2007). Peer-mediated social communication intervention: When clinical expertise informs treatment development and evaluation. *Topics in Language Disorders, 27*, 182–199.

Goldstein, H., & Wickstrom, S. (1986). Peer intervention effects on communicative interaction among handicapped and nonhandicapped preschoolers. *Journal of Applied Behavior Analysis, 19*, 209–214.

Grether, S. M., & Sickman, L. S. (2008). AAC and RTI: Building classroom-based strategies for every child in the classroom. *Seminars in Speech and Language, 29*, 155–163. doi:10.1055/s-2008-1079129.

Hendricks, D. R., & Wehman, P. (2009). Transition from school to adulthood for youth with autism spectrum disorders: Review and recommendations. *Focus on Autism & Other Developmental Disabilities, 24*, 77–88.

Hunt, P., Alwell, M., & Goetz, L. (1991). Establishing conversational exchanges with family and friends: Moving from training to meaningful communication. *The Journal of Special Education, 25*, 305–319.

Johnston, S. S., McDonnell, A. P., Nelson, C., & Magnavito, A. (2003). Teaching functional communication skills using augmentative and alternative communication in inclusive settings. *Journal of Early Intervention, 25*, 263–280.

Jonsson, A., Kristoffersson, L., Ferm, U., & Thunberg, G. (2011). The ComAlong communication boards: Parents' use and experiences of aided language stimulation. *Augmentative and Alternative Communication, 27*, 103–116. doi:10.3109/07434618.2011.580780.

Kent-Walsh, J., Binger, C., & Hasham, Z. (2010). Effects of parent instruction on the symbolic communication of children using augmentative and alternative communication during story-book reading. *American Journal of Speech-Language Pathology, 19*, 97–107. doi:10.1044/1058-0360(2010/09-0014).

Kent-Walsh, J., & Light, J. C. (2003). General education teachers' experiences with inclusion of students who use augmentative and alternative communication. *Augmentative and Alternative Communication, 19*, 104–124.

King, A. M., & Fahsl, A. J. (2012). Supporting social competence in children who use augmentative and alternative communication. *Teaching Exceptional Children, 45*, 42–49.

Light, J. (1997). "Let's go star fishing": Reflections on the contexts of language learning for children who use aided AAC. *Augmentative and Alternative Communication, 13*, 158–171. doi:10.1080/07434619712331277978.

Light, J. C., Binger, C., Agate, T. L., & Ramsay, K. N. (1999). Teaching partner-focused questions to individuals who use augmentative and alternative communication to enhance their communicative competence. *Journal of Speech, Language, and Hearing Research, 42*, 241–255.

Light, J., Dattilo, J., & English, J. (1992). Instructing facilitators to support the communication of people who use augmentative communication systems. *Journal of Speech & Hearing Research, 35*, 865–875.

Lilienfeld, M., & Alant, E. (2002). Attitudes of children toward an unfamiliar peer using an AAC device with and without voice output. *Augmentative and Alternative Communication, 18*, 91–101.

Lilienfeld, M., & Alant, E. (2005). The social interaction of an adolescent who uses AAC: The evaluation of a peer-training program. *Augmentative and Alternative Communication, 21*, 278–294. doi:10.1080/07434610500103467.

Marshall, J., & Goldbart, J. (2008). "Communication is everything I think." Parenting a child who needs augmentative and alternative communication (AAC). *International Journal of Language & Communication Disorders, 43*, 77–98.

Matson, J. L., Matson, M. L., & Rivet, T. T. (2007). Social-skills treatments for children with autism spectrum disorders. *Behavior Modification, 31*, 682–707.

McConkey, R., Truesdale-Kennedy, M., Crawford, H., McGreevy, E., Reavey, M., & Cassidy, A. (2010). Preschoolers with autism spectrum disorders: Evaluating the impact of a home-based intervention to promote their communication. *Early Child Development and Care, 180*, 299–315.

National Autism Center. (2009). *National standards report*. Randolph, MA: Author.

Nelson, C., McDonnell, A. P., Johnston, S. S., Crompton, A., & Nelson, A. R. (2007). Keys to play: A strategy to increase the social interactions of young children with autism and their typically developing peers. *Education and Training in Developmental Disabilities, 42*, 165–181.

Nunes, D., & Hanline, M. F. (2007). Enhancing the alternative and augmentative communication use of a child with autism through a parent-implemented naturalistic intervention. *International Journal of Disability, Development & Education, 54*, 177–197. doi:10.1080/10349120701330495.

Owen-DeSchryver, J. S., Carr, E. G., Cale, S. I., & Blakeley-Smith, A. (2008). Promoting social interactions between students with autism spectrum disorders and their peers in inclusive school settings. *Focus on Autism and Other Developmental Disabilities, 23*, 15–28.

Park, J. H., Alber-Morgan, S., & Cannella-Malone, H. (2011). Effects of mother-implemented picture exchange communication system (PECS) training on independent communicative behaviors of young children with autism spectrum disorders. *Topics in Early Childhood Special Education, 31*, 37–47.

Ratcliff, A. E., & Cress, C. J. (1999). Guidelines for enhancing reciprocal peer communication with adolescents who use augmentative/alternative communication. *Journal of Children's Communication Development, 20*, 25–35.

Romski, M., Sevcik, R. A., Adamson, L. B., Smith, A., Cheslock, M., & Bakeman, R. (2011). Parent perceptions of the language development of toddlers with developmental delays before and after participation in parent-coached language interventions. *American Journal of Speech-Language Pathology, 20*, 111–118. doi:10.1044/1058-0360(2011/09-0087).

Sainato, D. M., Goldstein, H., & Strain, P. S. (1992). Effects of self-evaluation on preschool children's use of social interaction strategies with their classmates with autism. *Journal of Applied Behavior Analysis, 25*, 127–141. doi:10.1901/jaba.1992.25-127.

Sawyer, L., Luiselli, J., Ricciardi, J., & Gower, J. (2005). Teaching a child with autism to share among peers in an integrated preschool classroom: Acquisition, maintenance, and social validation. *Education and Treatment of Children, 28*, 1–10.

Sigafoos, J., O'Reilly, M. F., Seely-York, S., Weru, J., Son, S. H., Green, V. A., & Lancioni, G. E. (2004). Transferring AAC intervention to the home. *Disability & Rehabilitation, 26*, 1330–1334. doi:10.1080/09638280412331280361.

Simpson, R. L., Ganz, J. B., & Mason, R. A. (2012). Social skills interventions and programming for learners with autism spectrum disorders. In D. Zager, M. L. Wehmeyer, & R. L. Simpson (Eds.), *Educating students with autism spectrum disorders: Research-based principles and practices*. New York: Routledge.

Smith, A. L., Romski, M. A., Sevcik, R. A., Adamson, L. B., & Bakeman, R. (2011). Parent stress and its relation to parent perceptions of communication following parent-coached language intervention. *Journal of Early Intervention, 33*, 135–150.

Strain, P. S. (1977). Effects of peer social initiations on withdrawn preschool children: Some training and generalization effects. *Journal of Abnormal Child Psychology, 5*, 445–455.

Strain, P. S., & Bovey, E. H. (2011). Randomized, controlled trial of the LEAP model of early intervention for young children with autism spectrum disorders. *Topics in Early Childhood Special Education, 31*, 133–154.

Strain, P. S., Kerr, M. M., & Ragland, E. U. (1979). Effects of peer-mediated social initiation and prompting/reinforcement procedures on the social behavior of autistic children. *Journal of Autism and Developmental Disorders, 9*, 41–54.

Strain, P. S., Shores, R. E., & Timm, M. A. (1977). Effects of peer social initiations of the behavior of withdrawn preschool children. *Journal of Applied Behavior Analysis, 10*, 289–298.

Thiemann, K. S., & Goldstein, H. (2004). Effects of peer training and written text cueing on social communication of school-age children with pervasive developmental disorder. *Journal of Speech, Language, and Hearing Research, 47*, 126–144.

Thunberg, G., Ahlsén, E., & Sandberg, A. D. (2009a). Interaction and use of speech-generating devices in the homes of children with autism spectrum disorders—An analysis of conversational topics. *Journal of Special Education Technology, 24*, 1–16.

Thunberg, G., Sandberg, A. D., & Ahlsén, E. (2009b). Speech-generating devices used at home by children with autism spectrum disorders: A preliminary assessment. *Focus on Autism and Other Developmental Disabilities, 24*, 104–114.

Trembath, D., Balandin, S., Togher, L., & Stancliffe, R. J. (2009). Peer-mediated teaching and augmentative and alternative communication for preschool-aged children with autism. *Journal of Intellectual & Developmental Disability, 34*, 173–186.

Trottier, N., Kamp, L., & Mirenda, P. (2011). Effects of peer-mediated instruction to teach use of speech-generating devices to students with autism in social game routines. *Augmentative and Alternative Communication, 27*, 26–39. doi:10.3109/07434618.2010.546810.

Chapter 7
Functional Communication Training with Aided AAC

Jennifer B. Ganz and Ee Rea Hong

What Is Functional Communication Training

As noted in Chap. 1, people with ASD and CCN frequently engage in challenging behavior, and providing AAC may reduce the need for these behaviors (Ganz et al. 2009; Sigafoos et al. 2008). Functional communication training (FCT) is an approach to addressing challenging behaviors that involves determining why the behavior is occurring (i.e., what function does the behavior serve) and teaching the individual a more acceptable mode of communicating to get his or her desired reinforcement than via the challenging behavior (Durand and Merges 2001). FCT is based on the idea that challenging behavior serves communicative purposes (Durand 1990). Although FCT does often involve AAC as the communication mode taught, it cannot be accurately described as an AAC system, because FCT is implemented to address challenging behaviors only (Durand and Merges 2001). That is, the research on FCT typically does not involve implementation of a comprehensive communication system, although some participants may already use aided AAC (Durand and Merges 2001). There are two key steps to implementing FCT. First, the interventionist conducts a functional behavior assessment (FBA) (Mancil 2006). Second, once the interventionist develops a hypothesis regarding the function of the behavior, or in some cases multiple functions of the behavior, he or she implements FCT. Details of each are provided below.

> **Scenario**
>
> Noah's special education teacher, Ms. Han, was concerned due to the frequency in which he engaged in high pitched shrieking. Although he was capable of independently participating in center activities in his kindergarten homeroom,

(continued)

J.B. Ganz, *Aided Augmentative Communication for Individuals with Autism Spectrum Disorders*, Autism and Child Psychopathology Series, DOI 10.1007/978-1-4939-0814-1_7, © Springer Science+Business Media New York 2014

(continued)

his kindergarten teacher, Mr. Kennard, noted that the shrieking was keeping him from fitting in with his classmates and, as a result, Mr. Kennard asked that Noah spend less time in his class, particularly during centers. Ms. Han asked if he would give her a week to observe and assess the situation before making any decisions, to which Mr. Kennard agreed.

Functional Behavior Assessment

An FBA includes a variety of direct and indirect observation tools that assist the practitioner in determining why the client is engaging in challenging behavior. These tools include interviewing the individual and caregivers, observing challenging behaviors using behavioral tools, using indirect tools such as behavioral checklists, and conducting experimental functional analyses (FAs) (Mancil 2006). Each of these components is discussed below, with particular attention to FAs. There have been a number of indirect (i.e., not direct observations) behavioral checklists developed over the last few decades that aim to determine the functions of challenging behavior. One, the *Questions About Behavioral Function* (QABF) (Matson et al. 1999; Matson and Vollmer 1995) has recently received attention in the literature as having high convergent validity with experimental FAs and with other behavioral checklists (Freeman et al. 2007; Paclawskyj et al. 2001). That is, the QABF has been found to result in a determination of a function of the behavior that closely matches other FBA checklists and the results of experimental FAs, including when evaluating challenging behaviors (Watkins and Rapp 2013) and stereotypic behaviors (Wilke et al. 2012; Zaja et al. 2011), and including with individuals with ASD. Further, the QABF has been found to have good test–retest reliability (Shogren and Rojahn 2003) and fair inter-rater reliability (Nicholson et al. 2006; Paclawskyj et al. 2000; Smith et al. 2012). In other words, when repeated over time, the QABF tends to have similar results each time, and different raters (e.g., teacher and educational assistant), including those with little behavioral training, have fair rates of agreement on their assessments of the client. The QABF also has appropriate internal consistency (Freeman et al. 2007; Paclawskyj et al. 2000; Shogren and Rojahn 2003), meaning that the subscale questions are strongly related. These indicators are among those that are considered to be critical when determining the usefulness of a chosen assessment.

Scenario

On Friday, Ms. Han asked Mr. Kennard and the class educational aide to complete a checklist and asked him to describe the behavior thoroughly and when they thought it occurred. The results of the QABF indicated that both "escape" from aversive attention and "tangible," or desire for preferred objects, were likely functions of Noah's shrieking. Specifically, the teacher and aide indicated that the shrieking seemed to occur most often when he was engaged in his favorite activities and another child came close, talked to him, or touched or took some of the materials with which he was working.

An experimental FA typically involves highly controlled testing a number of hypotheses regarding the possible function of a challenging behavior (Carr and Durand 1985). This often includes conditions to evaluate the role of preferred items, attention, desire for escape from aversive activities or items, and self-stimulation (e.g., stereotypy, repetitive motions thought to provide the individual with desired sensory stimulation) (Matson et al. 1999). Conditions that occur before or after the behavior are manipulated and data are collected in each condition to determine what triggers the highest instances of the challenging behavior (Wacker et al. 2013). These conditions are often repeated several times to confirm the hypothesis that one or more of the conditions trigger the behavior, or what are the primary functions of that particular challenging behavior. In some instances, FAs are sometimes conducted in less structured contexts, such as within natural environments (Mancil and Boman 2010). For more information on how to conduct FAs, readers are advised to seek training in behavior analysis. Such training, specifically related to conducting FAs, may be provided in workshops, online trainings, or as part of university degree or certification programs. Experimental FAs are not typically performed by lay people or professionals who do not have behavioral training.

Often, though not always, FCT interventions include only the experimental FA component of the FBA. In a few cases, FCT has been implemented with other components of FBA and excluding an FA. When determining whether to conduct an experimental FA or use a checklist, there are several factors to consider. One, FAs are time consuming (Paclawskyj et al. 2000). Depending on the number of contexts evaluated, FAs may take up to several hours to complete. The QABF checklist, however, takes approximately 20 m to administer, allowing clinicians to save time and resources for conducting experimental FAs only in extreme cases (Paclawskyj et al. 2000; Wilke et al. 2012). Two, FAs are best conducted by individuals with advanced training (Paclawskyj et al. 2000). Thus, teachers and other educational professional in most settings may not be equipped to conduct FAs, while a checklist may be more manageable. Three, checklists may be better at evaluating behavioral functions for behaviors that occur at low frequencies, thus are less detectable in experimental FAs that reflect only a short period of time and limited conditions (Paclawskyj et al. 2001), although low frequency behaviors may indeed be severe and harmful. Because of these reasons, it may be feasible in most cases to complete a QABF first and continue to an experimental FA only if the QABF is inconclusive or in particularly severe cases, in which case, a consultant with extensive behavioral knowledge and experience may be called in.

Scenario

On Monday, Ms. Han watched as center time began and took narrative notes. Using a visual choice board, Noah selected painting as his activity. He willingly walked over to an easel and the class educational aide helped him put on a smock, choose paint colors, and set up a sheet of paper and brushes. Noah quietly waited. When it was set up, he began painting while humming quietly. About 5 min after he began painting, another boy, Hunter, walked over to the easel, stood within a few inches of Noah and touched Noah's paper saying, "I like the green part." At the moment Hunter touched his paper, Noah started making an ear-piercing screech and Hunter immediately walked away, after which Noah went back to humming and painting. After observing and noting four other similar circumstances when Noah was painting, coloring with markers, and looking at books, Ms. Han decided to conduct an FA.

Although Ms. Han thought that Noah was shrieking to avoid attention, it was not clear to her if it was only due to attention from peers or if Noah was trying to maintain access to his preferred materials and thought that if other children touched the materials, they might take them away. In the interview, Mr. Kennard had noted that Noah had three brothers and a sister and that his mother had said he also shrieked when one of his siblings took one of the toys with which he was playing. So, Ms. Han decided to conduct an FA to test four conditions. Each condition was conducted for 5 min during recess, so the other children would not be in the room, lessening the chance for Noah to be ostracized by the high occurrences of challenging behavior often seen during FAs. Noah was in the classroom for each condition, engaged in painting or coloring with markers. Data were collected during each 10-s interval; Ms. Han marked "+" or "−" to indicate whether or not the shrieking had occurred during that 10-s interval.

The first condition was an "Alone" condition, during which Noah was alone in the room, while Ms. Han observed from just outside the door, where she could see and hear Noah, but Noah did not see her. The second condition was an "Escape Attention" condition; approximately every 30 s, Ms. Han walked over to Noah and stood within 6 in. of him and commented on his artwork. Contingent upon Noah shrieking, Ms. Han would stop talking and move about 10 ft away until 30 s had passed. The third condition, "Access Tangibles," was evaluated by Ms. Han walking to Noah every 30 s and taking one of the markers or paint brushes. Contingent upon shrieking, she would place the item back on the table or easel. The final condition, "Escape, plus Access," involved a combination of the second and third conditions, during which Ms. Han both talked to Noah and picked up one of his items. The data in Fig. 7.1 illustrate Ms. Han's findings.

These data indicate that, although the behavior was about equally as frequent in the Access Tangibles and the Escape, plus Access conditions, because it did not occur during the Escape Attention condition, it was likely that the behavior most often occurred due to other children touching his items.

(continued)

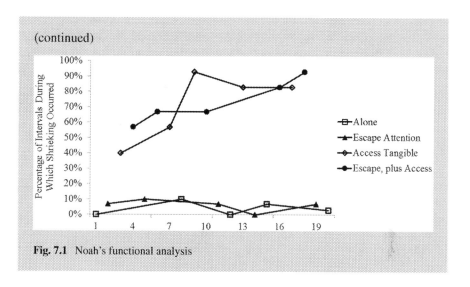

Fig. 7.1 Noah's functional analysis

Functional Communication Training

FCT involves implementation of instruction in the new communication mode to replace a challenging behavior (Durand and Merges 2001). Recommended steps and components in implementation of FCT are described below.

Step 1: Selecting a communication mode. Following the FBA, once a hypothesis regarding the function, or multiple functions, of the challenging behavior is obtained, an alternative, more prosocial, communication behavior is selected for intervention. FCT can be used with any communication mode, including verbalizations, sign language, and aided AAC (Mancil 2006). Chapter 3 provides information regarding assessments for use in determining whether or not AAC is a reasonable choice for a particular client and detailed information regarding selecting an appropriate AAC mode. Schieltz et al. (2011) suggested that incorporating the use of aided AAC into FCT interventions may decrease the response effort required. That is, even if children have some ability to speak, destructive or disruptive behavior may require less effort than speaking, which may not be true for aided AAC devices that may require simple, quick motor movements to activate, thus quickly accessing reinforcement. Further, the concrete and visual qualities of the device may serve as a signaled reinforcer, or a sign that reinforcers are available (Schieltz et al. 2011). Harding and colleagues (2009) have noted that the use of concrete visual supports, such as those provided by AAC, may be helpful, even with individuals with ASD who have some speech.

Durand and Merges (2001) provided four areas of consideration when selecting a communication mode when implementing FCT. First, implementers should consider "response match" (Durand and Merges 2001). That is, the new communication behavior should fulfill the same function as that identified through the FBA.

For example, if the person pushes work off of her desk to avoid tasks that are too frustrating, the new communication skill should provide a more effective means to communicate that the task should stop. Although the implementers may feel that this is teaching the person a means to avoid doing work, once the challenging behavior is under control, one could implement a means of offering reinforcement for completing tasks and build up tolerance for such tasks slowly, rather than continuing to make little progress having the person complete her work.

Second, implementers should consider "response mastery" (Durand and Merges 2001). Several factors influence how well the target individual will master the new communicative skill. One factor is how successful the communicative behavior is in gaining the desired response from others. That is, if the person is taught to use her SGD to state, "*no thank you*" when presented with a difficult task, but the classroom staff continue to insist she work on the task immediately, that individual will not be receiving reinforcement for using the new behavior and will be unlikely to master it. Another factor is the efficiency of the new communicative behavior (Durand and Merges 2001). In other words, does the new behavior require manageable physical effort and does it result in sufficient access to reinforcement? If the individual has difficulty talking and the new behavior requires a four-word spoken phrase, he or she is unlikely to master that communicative behavior. If the new behavior is initially rewarded every time it is used, it is more likely to be mastered than if it is infrequently rewarded. Another factor in mastery of the skill is its social acceptability (Durand and Merges 2001). That is, if the communicative intent or mode is unacceptable to the stakeholders in the person's environment, they are unlikely to reinforce the behavior; thus, their interests and considerations should be paramount. Chapter 4 provides information regarding collaborating with and garnering input from interdisciplinary stakeholders. Finally, implementers should consider how recognizable the communicative behavior is to those who will likely respond to the person (Durand and Merges 2001). For example, if the person can speak, but much of his speech is unrecognizable, the communicative attempts are likely to lead to frustration on the part of the person with CCN and the communicative partners. Thus, an AAC mode may be more appropriate, particularly when addressing challenging behaviors, if it results in a clear, consistent communication.

Third, the implementers should address "response milieu" (Durand and Merges 2001). Environments that allow the individual to have choices regarding his or her daily activities are likely to promote learning of and use of new communication skills. For example, providing opportunities to select which task to do first, what foods to eat, and what recreational activities to engage in will encourage the person to have control and use his or her communication skills (Durand and Merges 2001). Further, Durand and Merges recommend significant collaboration between general education teachers, special education teachers, family members, and other key stakeholders when implementing FCT; such collaborative approaches are discussed in Chap. 4. Further information related to teaching for generalization of skills across contexts is addressed below. The fourth area that Durand and Merges recommend that implementers consider is the consequence for the person engaging in challenging behaviors, which is discussed further below, related to extinction.

Step 2: Teaching the client to use the new communication mode. The next step in implementation of FCT is teaching the replacement communicative behavior to the individual with ASD. A variety of instructional strategies may be used to teach the new communicative behavior to replace prior challenging behaviors. This may involve some discrete trial instruction, but naturalistic strategies that involve use of communication in the actual settings and contexts in which the skills are needed are recommended (Durand and Merges 2001). Further, the implementer should have some knowledge and skill in selecting and implementing language instruction. Chapters 5 and 6 provide detailed recommendations and resources for teaching communication skills to individuals with ASD who have CCN within naturalistic contexts.

Step 3: Reinforcement contingent upon the desired communicative behavior. A key component to the success of FCT is providing reinforcement contingent upon the individual exhibiting the targeted communication behavior (Snell et al. 2006), which teaches the person that the new prosocial mode is a more effective means of gaining access to reinforcement than the prior method. Although parents and educators may be uncomfortable rewarding some communication behaviors, such as work avoidance, in order to decrease the challenging behavior, the individual should first be taught the appropriate communicative replacement behavior (Mancil 2006). To ensure that behavior is mastered, it must be reinforced at a high rate initially. Later, a delay may be introduced. For example, the person may later be told that he or she must first do a very small amount of work before receiving a break, which would then slowly be increased once the communicative behavior was demonstrated to have been maintained over the fading of immediate reinforcement.

Component A: Extinction of challenging behaviors. Extinction of the challenging behavior that previously was reinforced is typically implemented at the same time as FCT (Falcomata and Wacker 2013; Harding et al. 2009). That is, challenging behaviors are no longer reinforced or rewarded with attention, access to preferred items, or escape from aversive activities. However, in some cases, extinction was not a component of intervention, but the FCT intervention was still successful (O'Neill and Sweetland-Baker 2001). One key to successful implementation of FCT is that the newly learned communicative behavior becomes more effective in allowing the person with CCN to access reinforcement (Durand and Merges 2001). Thus, when the new skill is rewarded while the challenging behavior is ignored, the new skill is more likely to be maintained. However, in the event that the challenging behavior is dangerous to the individual or others or results in severe property damage, people must be protected from harm; thus, extinction implementation must be decided on a case-by-case basis (Durand and Merges 2001).

Component B: Teaching for generalization. FCT instruction should be implemented with systematic instruction taking place to ensure generalization (Falcomata and Wacker 2013). Generalization of learning of new skills means that skills learned in one context, with one instructor, in one setting, and with one set of materials are also able to be performed in other contexts, with other people, in other settings, and with other materials (Mancil and Boman 2010). Generalization is of particular concern when working with individuals with ASD as they often demonstrate stimulus over-selectivity; that is, they often focus on single or few aspects of stimuli present when learning, thus acquire new skills only in the particular contexts in which they are taught and only with a particular person or in a particular setting without understanding that the same skills may be performed in other contexts (Mancil 2006). Instructors should plan for systematically addressing generalization across contexts, items, people, vocabulary, and communicative functions (Falcomata and Wacker 2013).

To promote generalization, instruction should be provided via a variety of contexts (Stokes and Osnes 1989). That is, instruction in the new communication behavior should explicitly be taught with a number of instructors, with a number of materials, in a number of settings, and in a number of tasks or contexts. Moreover, all natural settings in which the target communication skills will be used should be identified for intervention (Mancil and Boman 2010). People with ASD typically do not spontaneously generalize skills across contexts; thus, interventionists must consider all the potential settings and contexts in which the new skill may be used. For example, if a person with CCN is being taught to respond to a question asking him to choose among several food items, interventionists should consider all contexts in which choices may be offered, such as at restaurants, during free time at home, and when choosing what to wear for the day. In such a case, the interventionist should target all of the possible contexts necessary and vocabulary needed in each case.

All people who may be communicative partners, including family members and peers, should be included in intervention (Mancil and Boman 2010). This is critical to ensure that people with ASD and CCN do not limit their AAC use to the person who provided them with initial instruction only. Further, the interventionist should explain to each communicative partner the nature of the communication and what the expected response is. For instance, it should be explained to the paraprofessional that in the initial instructional phase, a student should be reinforced with play items every time they are asked for, with the understanding that, once the behavior is mastered, the student will be taught to wait or complete work before receiving the reward (Mancil and Boman 2010).

FCT instruction should, as any instruction with an eye toward generalization should, incorporate "recruitment of natural reinforcers" (Stokes and Osnes 1989). That is, instructors should teach new communication modes that are likely to be reinforced in natural contexts. For example, if a child who throws the computer keyboard on the floor when it is not turned on when he goes to play a game is taught to ask for help by selecting an icon that says "*I need help!*" This behavior would likely result in someone helping him gain access to the game. Teaching behaviors that are likely to be reinforced by people other than those who provided the initial instruction and for a variety of contexts (e.g., when the microwave is not working properly, when the smartphone's battery has run down) increases the likelihood that if the client engages in these behaviors elsewhere, he or she will likely also be reinforced in those contexts. Thus, the client would be motivated to continue to use that behavior. In many cases, it may be beneficial to provide instruction to others who will interact with the client so they also reinforce the new communicative behaviors (Falcomata and Wacker 2013).

Scenario

Because Noah's shrieking appeared to serve as a protest against others touching his project materials, Ms. Han and Mr. Kennard decided to implement an FCT intervention. Noah already used a tablet computer AAC app to request food at snack and lunch time, math manipulatives during math small group instruction, and materials at center time. The app was programed with matrices of 6–8 icons for each activity and each icon, when selected, would emit a short phrase, such as "*marker please*." The teachers or aide would select the correct page at the beginning of each activity. Because Noah was already able to use his app consistently and independently for some activities, the teachers incorporated a new icon on the page for each center activity (i.e., painting center, coloring center, and book center) that produced the phrase, "*don't touch*" when selected.

Initially, the teachers taught Noah to use the new icon with them when the classroom was otherwise empty. They extinguished the shrieking by ignoring it. At the same time, they taught him to use the new icon by letting him get started with one of the center activities, moving close while reaching toward the items he was using, and immediately modeling by touching the icon, saying, "don't touch," and backing away. When he did not begin using the icon with a model alone, the teachers went through the same sequence but replaced the model with a physical prompt to help him touch the new icon. They were quickly able to fade the prompt. When Noah consistently and independently used the icon and ceased shrieking, they introduced two classmates when the classroom was otherwise empty. The teachers stood nearby and quickly prompted Noah if he began to shriek when the other children got close. Eventually, Noah was able to use the icon independently during regular center time, with little shrieking. Later, the teachers worked with Noah's family to ensure he was using the same symbol at home, though it was on a choice board in the living room where he played video games, to communicate to his big brother to let him play his game alone.

Research on FCT

Although the research supporting FCT is wide (Falcomata and Wacker 2013; Kurtz et al. 2011; Mirenda 1997; Mancil 2006), because this book focuses on ASD, the FCT research that is summarized below focuses only on people with ASD. The first table covers research involving FCT research with people with ASD who could talk or used unaided AAC (see Table 7.1) while the second table includes only studies with people with ASD and CCN who used some form of aided AAC within the studies (see Table 7.2).

Table 7.1 FCT with people with ASD, excluding AAC

Author(s) (year)	N	Age range (years)	Diagnoses[a]	Participants reported to have some speech	Communication mode(s)[b]	Study design[c]	Intervention summary	Maintenance or generalization assessed	Results summary	Type of FBA
Braithwaite and Richdale (2000)	1	7	AU	Y	SP	SCD-F	Behavioral strategies (verbal prompts, delay of reinforcement, shaping)	N	Increased in use of phrases and decreased in self-injurious and aggressive behaviors	FBA without FA
Falcomata et al. (2012b)	1	8	AU	N	SP	SCD	Behavioral strategies (gestural prompt, reinforcement, extinction)	N	Increased rates of manding and decreased in challenging behaviors	Analogue FA
Falcomata et al. (2013a)	2	7, 12	AU	Y	SP	SCD	Behavioral strategies (delay of reinforcement, verbal prompt, gestural prompt, extinction)	N	Increased rates of manding and decreased in challenging behaviors	Analogue FA
Falcomata et al. (2012a)	2	8	PDD/HFA, AU	N	SP	SCD	Behavioral strategies (verbal prompt, physical prompt, graduated prompting procedure, reinforcement, fading)	N	Increased rates of manding and decreased in challenging behaviors	Analogue FA
Falcomata et al. (2013b)	3	2.2–4.4	DD, AU	Y	MS	SCD-F	Behavioral strategies (vocal prompt, physical prompt)	Y	Increased in use of sign language and generalized to different signs and decreased in destructive behaviors	Analogue FA
Gerhardt et al. (2003)	1	18	AU	N	MS	CS	Behavioral strategies (reinforcement)	N	Increased in use of sign language and decreased in aggressive behaviors	Analogue FA/FBA without FA
Gibson et al. (2010)	1	4	AU	Y	MS	SCD	Behavioral strategies (modeling, prompt)	N	Increased in use of sign language and decreased in elopement	FBA without FA/Brief FA
Lalli et al. (1995)	2	13, 15	AU/ID	Y	SP	SCD	Behavioral strategies (extinction, modeled prompt)	N	Increased in independent verbalizations and decreased in self-injurious behaviors	Brief FA
Ross (2002)	3	9–14.10	AU	Y	SP	SCD-F	Behavioral strategies (time delay, modeling)	N	Increased in correct response and conversational exchanges and decreased in faulty responses	Analogue FA/FBA without FA

[a]*AU* autism, autistic disorder, early infantile autism, *DD* developmental delay, developmental disability, *ID* intellectual disability, mental retardation, *PDD/HFA* pervasive developmental disorder, not otherwise specified, Asperger syndrome, high functioning autism, "autism spectrum disorder" without a specific diagnosis, *SD* sensory disability, *OTH* other disabilities (e.g., chromosomal abnormalities); diagnosis definitions listed here reflect the terms used in the original articles, though may be outdated

[b]*MS* manual sign language, *PE* picture-exchange system (including the Picture Exchange Communication System), *SGD-SO* speech-generating device or voice output communication aid with single-switch or changeable overlays, *SGD-DD* speech-generating device or voice output communication aid with dynamic displays, such as computer screens, *SP* speech

[c]*CS* case study, narrative description, *G* group study, *SCD* robust single-case design, *SCD-F* single-case design with significant design flaws

Table 7.2 FCT with people with ASD and aided AAC as the communication mode

Author(s) (year)	N	Age range (years)	Diagnoses[a]	Participants reported to have some speech	Communication mode(s)[b]	Study design[c]	Intervention summary	Maintenance or generalization assessed	Results summary	Type of FBA
Buckley and Newchok (2005)	1	7	AU	Y	PE	SCD-F	Behavioral strategies (reinforcement, physical prompt, extinction)	N	Increased in picture exchanges and decreased in aggression	Analogue FA
Casey and Merical (2006)	1	11	AU	N	PE/SP	SCD	Behavioral strategies (verbal prompt)	Y	Increased in verbalization and number of picture touch	Brief FA
Falcomata et al. (2010)	1	5	AU	Y	PE	SCD-F	Behavioral strategies (physical guidance, Fading)	N	Increased in number of card touch and decreased in rates of elopement	Analogue FA
Fisher et al. (2005)	2	13, 14	AU/ID	N	PE	SCD-F	Behavioral strategies (verbal prompt, modeled prompt, reinforcement)	N	Decreased in destructive behaviors. Both participants chose positive reinforcement over negative reinforcement	Analogue FA
Hines and Simonsen (2008)	1	3.5	AU	N	PE	SCD-F	Behavioral strategies (verbal prompt, reinforcement, fading)	Y	Increased in card use and decreased in disruptive vocalization across phases	FBA without FA
Martin et al. (2005)	1	10	AU	N	PE	SCD-F	Behavioral strategies (physical prompt, error correction)	N	Increased in picture use and decreased in problem behaviors (i.e., pushing away)	FBA without FA
Olive et al. (2008)	1	4	AU	Y	SGD-SO	SCD	Behavioral strategies (physical prompt, graduated guidance, prompting, gestural prompt, verbal prompt, fading)	N	Increased in number of requests and correct use of pronouns and decreased in challenging behaviors	FBA without FA/Analogue FA
O'Neill and Sweetland-Baker (2001)	2	6, 15	AU/ID	N	PE	SCD-F	Behavioral strategies (gestural and physical Prompt, fading)	Y	Increased in unprompted requests and decreased in disruptive behaviors. Mixed results in untrained tasks	Analogue FA

(continued)

Table 7.2 (continued)

Author(s) (year)	N	Age range (years)	Diagnoses[a]	Participants reported to have some speech	Communication mode(s)[b]	Study design[c]	Intervention summary	Maintenance or generalization assessed	Results summary	Type of FBA
Schieltz et al. (2011)	4	2.3–3.11	AU/ID/DD	Y	SGD-SO	SCD	Behavioral strategies (physical prompt, Modeling, reinforcement, fading)	N	Decreased in targeted disruptive and non-targeted disruptive behaviors	Analogue FA
Sigafoos and Meikle (1996)	2	1.8–3.4	AU/ID	Y	PE	SCD-F	Behavioral strategies (physical and verbal prompts, modeling)	Y	Increased in card use and decreased in disruptive behaviors	Analogue FA
Volkert et al. (2009)	1	9	AU/DD	Y	PE	SCD	Behavioral strategies (physical prompt with a progressive prompt delay)	Y	Increased in use of card and decreased in problem behaviors	Analogue FA
Wacker et al. (2013)	20	2.5–6.8	AU/PDD/HFA	Y	PE/SGD-SO	SCD	Behavioral strategies (prompt)	N	All the parents accurately implemented FA	Analogue FA
Wu et al. (2010)	1	17	AU	N	SGD-SO	CS	Behavioral strategies (prompt)	N	Increased in independent requests and decreased in loud vocalizations	FBA without FA/Brief FA

[a]AU autism, autistic disorder, early infantile autism, DD developmental delay, developmental disability, ID intellectual disability, mental retardation, PDD/HFA pervasive developmental disorder, not otherwise specified, Asperger syndrome, high functioning autism, "autism spectrum disorder" without a specific diagnosis, SD sensory disability, OTH other disabilities (e.g., chromosomal abnormalities); diagnosis definitions listed here reflect the terms used in the original articles, though they may be outdated

[b]MS manual sign language, PE picture-exchange system (including the Picture Exchange Communication System), SGD-SO speech-generating device or voice output communication aid with single-switch or changeable overlays, SGD-DD speech-generating device or voice output communication aid with dynamic displays, such as computer screens, SP speech

[c]CS case study, narrative description, G group study, SCD robust single-case design, SCD-F single-case design with significant design flaws

FCT Research with People with ASD

Most of the research supporting the use of FCT with people with autism has included young participants (Mancil 2006). In particular, preschool aged children with ASD have been frequently included as participants in FCT studies (Falcomata et al. 2013b; Gibson et al. 2010). In a small number of studies, older children or adults with ASD were studied (Lalli et al. 1995). FCT has been implemented with individuals with a wide range of language and cognitive functioning (Mancil 2006). That is, it has been used with people with CCN (Falcomata et al. 2013b) as well as people with age-appropriate speech skills and those with some functional speech (Braithwaite and Richdale 2000; Falcomata et al. 2012a), although more often has been implemented with children and youth with communication deficits. Further, participants for whom FCT has been successful have included those with ASD and ID (Braithwaite and Richdale 2000; Lalli et al. 1995). In some cases, FCT has been successfully implemented with individuals with ASD to treat multiple communicative functions, such as attention-seeking and tangible reinforcement (Falcomata et al. 2012b, 2013a).

Most of the FCT interventions have been implemented by researchers rather than natural communication partners, such as teachers, and have often been implemented in separate or clinical settings (Mancil 2006). However, one recent FCT study is of particular interest because it involved the use of distance technology and family members as implementers. Wacker et al. (2013) recently conducted a study involving implementing FCT via telehealth with parents of 17 young children with ASD and challenging behaviors as implementers at regional clinics set up for videoconferencing. Behavior consultants provided videoconferencing instructions to parents and "family navigators" who assisted the parents, but had no prior behavioral training. Results were positive and comparable with those of in vivo implementation of parent-implemented FCT. Cost analyses indicated significant savings for telehealth-provided FCT versus in vivo.

Overall, studies involving implementation of FCT with individuals with ASD have had positive results. However, a number of these studies have used weak research designs (Braithwaite and Richdale 2000), had inconclusive evidence (Falcomata et al. 2013b), or procedures involving data collection or prompt fading are not clear (Gibson et al. 2010), making it difficult to confidently interpret their results. Further, generalization was infrequently evaluated in FCT studies with people with ASD.

FCT Research Involving AAC with People with ASD

There is a limited quantity of studies involving the implementation of FCT with people with ASD via the use of an aided AAC communication mode. The range of individuals in such studies has ranged from preschool (Hines and Simonsen 2008; Olive et al. 2008; Schieltz et al. 2011) to elementary-aged individuals (Casey and Merical 2006; Leon et al. 2013; Sigafoos and Meikle 1996) and middle and high school children (Fisher et al. 2005; O'Neill and Sweetland-Baker 2001); few studies have investigated the use of AAC to address behavior in adults (Ganz et al. 2012a, b; Walker and Snell 2013). Studies in this area have included the use of exchange-based AAC (Casey and Merical 2006; Fisher et al. 2005; Leon et al. 2013; Martin et al. 2005), picture point systems (Falcomata et al. 2010; Sigafoos and Meikle 1996), and speech-generating devices (Olive et al. 2008; Schieltz et al. 2011; Wacker et al. 2013). In this population, FCT has been successfully used via aided AAC to address attention-seeking behaviors (Olive et al. 2008), tangible motivated behaviors (Sigafoos and Meikle 1996), and self-stimulation seeking (Leon et al. 2013). These interventions have resulted in decreases in stereotypy (Falcomata et al. 2010), elopement, aggression (Buckley and Newchok 2005; Leon et al. 2013), and self-injury (Schieltz et al. 2011). Recently, Walker and Snell (2013) conducted a meta-analysis of the effects of AAC on challenging behavior. They found that there were moderate effects on individuals with ASD. Overall, studies involving all diagnostic categories that involved FCT had statistically significantly better effects related to decreases in challenging behavior than those involving PECS implementation, although both had moderate effects.

Conclusions

FCT is implemented to address challenging behaviors, not primarily to provide individuals with CCN with a means of functional communication (Durand and Merges 2001). However, FCT may be incorporated into existing communication systems as both a method of addressing behavior and teaching new communication skills. While AAC protocols often begin with instruction in requesting objects, the FCT literature may provide an impetus to teach other communication functions, including asking for help, protesting, and requesting attention. There is limited literature on the use of FCT for people with ASD who use AAC; clearly more research in this area is needed, perhaps linking FCT with comprehensive AAC instruction. It may be that incorporating FCT into AAC instruction may provide motivation for individuals with ASD to communicate because they are often highly motivated when frustrated. Although challenging behavior itself is not a criterion for an ASD diagnosis (APA 2013), because many people with ASD have significant communication challenges that may lead to a reliance on challenging behavior to communicate, FCT provides a means to both address challenging behavior and teach socially appropriate communication (Durand and Merges 2001).

References

American Psychiatric Association (APA). (2013). *Diagnostic and statistical manual* (5th ed.). Washington, DC: Author.

Braithwaite, K. L., & Richdale, A. L. (2000). Functional communication training to replace challenging behaviors across two behavioral outcomes. *Behavioral Interventions, 15*, 21–36.

Buckley, S. D., & Newchok, D. K. (2005). Differential impact of response effort within a response chain on use of mands in a student with autism. *Research in Developmental Disabilities, 26*, 77–85. doi:10.1016/j.ridd.2004.07.004.

Carr, E. G., & Durand, V. M. (1985). Reducing behavior problems through functional communication training. *Journal of Applied Behavior Analysis, 18*, 111–126.

Casey, S. D., & Merical, C. L. (2006). The use of functional communication training without additional treatment procedures in an inclusive school setting. *Behavioral Disorders, 32*, 46–54.

Durand, V. M. (1990). *Severe behavior problems: A functional communication training approach.* New York: Guilford.

Durand, V. M., & Merges, E. (2001). Functional communication training: A contemporary behavior analytic intervention for problem behaviors. *Focus on Autism and Other Developmental Disabilities, 16*(110–119), 136.

Falcomata, T. S., Muething, C. S., Gainey, S., Hoffman, K., & Fragale, C. (2013a). Further evaluations of functional communication training and chained schedules of reinforcement to treat multiple functions of challenging behavior. *Behavior Modification, 37*, 723–746. doi:10.1177/0145445513500785.

Falcomata, T. S., Roane, H. S., Feeney, B. J., & Stephenson, K. M. (2010). Assessment and treatment of elopement maintained by access to stereotypy. *Journal of Applied Behavior Analysis, 43*, 513–517.

Falcomata, T. S., Roane, H. S., Muething, C. S., Stephenson, K. M., & Ing, A. D. (2012a). Functional communication training and chained schedules of reinforcement to treat challenging behavior maintained by terminations of activity interruptions. *Behavior Modification, 36*, 630–649. doi:10.1177/0145445511433821.

Falcomata, T. S., & Wacker, D. P. (2013). On the use of strategies for programming generalization during functional communication training: A review of the literature. *Journal of Developmental and Physical Disabilities, 25*, 5–15. doi:10.1007/s10882-012-9311-3.

Falcomata, T. S., Wacker, D. P., Ringdahl, J. E., Vinquist, K., & Dutt, A. (2013b). An evaluation of generalization of mands during functional communication training. *Journal of Applied Behavior Analysis, 46*, 444–454. doi:10.1002/jaba.37.

Falcomata, T., White, P., Muething, C., & Fragale, C. (2012b). A functional communication training and chained schedule procedure to treat challenging behavior with multiple functions. *Journal of Developmental and Physical Disabilities, 24*, 529–538. doi:10.1007/s10882-012-9287-z.

Fisher, W. W., Adelinis, J. D., Volkert, V. M., Keeney, K. M., Neidert, P. L., & Hovanetz, A. (2005). Assessing preferences for positive and negative reinforcement during treatment of destructive behavior with functional communication training. *Research in Developmental Disabilities, 26*, 153–168. doi:10.1016/j.ridd.2004.01.007.

Freeman, K. A., Walker, M., & Kaufman, J. (2007). Psychometric properties of the Questions About Behavioral Function Scale in a child sample. *American Journal on Mental Retardation, 112*, 122–129. doi:10.1352/0895-8017(2007)112[122:PPOTQA]2.0.CO;2.

Ganz, J. B., Davis, J. L., Lund, E. M., Goodwyn, F. D., & Simpson, R. L. (2012a). Meta-analysis of PECS with individuals with ASD: Investigation of targeted versus non-targeted outcomes, participant characteristics, and implementation phase. *Research in Developmental Disorders, 33*, 406–418. doi:10.1016/j.ridd.2011.09.023.

Ganz, J. B., Earles-Vollrath, T. L., Heath, A. K., Parker, R., Rispoli, M. J., & Duran, J. (2012b). A meta-analysis of single case research studies on aided augmentative and alternative communication systems with individuals with autism spectrum disorders. *Journal of Autism and Developmental Disorders, 42*, 60–74. doi:10.1007/s10803-011-1212-2.

Ganz, J. B., Parker, R., & Benson, J. (2009). Impact of the Picture Exchange Communication System: Effects on communication and collateral effects on maladaptive behaviors. *Augmentative and Alternative Communication, 25*, 250–261. doi:10.3109/07434610903381111.

Gerhardt, P. F., Weiss, M. J., & Delmolino, L. (2003). Treatment of severe aggression in an adolescent with autism. *The Behavior Analyst Today, 4*, 386–394.

Gibson, J. L., Pennington, R. C., Stenhoff, D. M., & Hopper, J. S. (2010). Using desktop videoconferencing to deliver interventions to a preschool student with autism. *Topics in Early Childhood Special Education, 29*, 214–225.

Harding, J. W., Wacker, D. P., Berg, W. K., Winborn-Kemmerer, L., Lee, J. F., & Ibrahimovic, M. (2009). Analysis of multiple manding topographies during functional communication training. *Education & Treatment of Children, 32*, 21–36.

Hines, E., & Simonsen, B. (2008). The effects of picture icons on behavior for a young student with autism. *Beyond Behavior, 18*, 9–17.

Kurtz, P. F., Boelter, E. W., Jarmolowicz, D. P., Chin, M. D., & Hagopian, L. P. (2011). An analysis of functional communication training as an empirically supported treatment for problem behavior displayed by individuals with intellectual disabilities. *Research in Developmental Disabilities, 32*, 2935–2942. doi:10.1016/j.ridd.2011.05.009.

Lalli, J. S., Casey, S., & Kates, K. (1995). Reducing escape behavior and increasing task completion with functional communication training, extinction, and response chaining. *Journal of Applied Behavior Analysis, 28*, 261–268.

Leon, Y., Lazarchick, W. N., Rooker, G. W., & Deleon, I. G. (2013). Assessment of problem behavior evoked by disruption of ritualistic toy arrangements in a child with autism. *Journal of Applied Behavior Analysis, 46*, 507–511. doi:10.1002/jaba.41.

Mancil, G. R. (2006). Functional communication training: A review of the literature related to children with autism. *Education & Training in Developmental Disabilities, 41*, 213–224.

Mancil, G. R., & Boman, M. (2010). Functional communication training in the classroom: A guide for success. *Preventing School Failure, 54*, 238–246.

Martin, C. A., Drasgow, E., Halle, J. W., & Brucker, J. M. (2005). Teaching a child with autism and severe language delays to reject: Direct and indirect effects of functional communication training. *Educational Psychology, 25*, 287–304.

Matson, J. L., Bamburg, J. W., & Cherry, K. E. (1999). A validity study on the Questions About Behavioral Function (QABF) Scale: Predicting treatment success for self-injury, aggression, and stereotypies. *Research in Developmental Disabilities, 20*, 163–175. doi:10.1016/S0891-4222(98)00039-0.

Matson, J. L., & Vollmer, T. R. (1995). *User's guide: Questions About Behavioral Function (QABF)*. Baton Rouge, LA: Scientific Publishers.

Mirenda, P. (1997). Supporting individuals with challenging behavior through functional communication training and AAC: Research review. *Augmentative and Alternative Communication, 13*, 207–225.

Nicholson, J., Konstantinidi, E., & Furniss, F. (2006). On some psychometric properties of the Questions About Behavioral Function (QABF) Scale. *Research in Developmental Disabilities, 27*, 337–352. doi:10.1016/j.ridd.2005.04.001.

O'Neill, R. E., & Sweetland-Baker, M. (2001). Brief report: An assessment of stimulus generalization and contingency effects in functional communication training with two students with autism. *Journal of Autism & Developmental Disorders, 31*, 235–240.

Olive, M. L., Lang, R. B., & Davis, T. N. (2008). An analysis of the effects of functional communication and a voice output communication aid for a child with autism spectrum disorder. *Research in Autism Spectrum Disorders, 2*, 223–236.

Paclawskyj, T. R., Matson, J. L., Rush, K. S., Smalls, Y., & Vollmer, T. R. (2000). Questions About Behavioral Function (QABF): A behavioral checklist for functional assessment of aberrant behavior. *Research in Developmental Disabilities, 21*, 223–229. doi:10.1016/S0891-4222(00)00036-6.

Paclawskyj, T. R., Matson, J. L., Rush, K. S., Smalls, Y., & Vollmer, T. R. (2001). Assessment of the convergent validity of the Questions About Behavioral Function Scale with analogue functional analysis and the motivation assessment scale. *Journal of Intellectual Disability Research, 45*, 484–494. doi:10.1046/j.1365-2788.2001.00364.x.

Ross, D. E. (2002). Replacing faulty conversational exchanges for children with autism by establishing a functionally equivalent alternative response. *Education and Training in Mental Retardation and Developmental Disabilities, 37*, 343–362.

Schieltz, K. M., Wacker, D. P., Harding, J. W., Berg, W. K., Lee, J. F., Padilla Dalmau, Y. C., … Ibrahimovi, M. (2011). Indirect effects of functional communication training on non-targeted disruptive behavior. *Journal of Behavioral Education, 20*, 15–32. doi: 10.1007/s10864-011-9119-8.

Shogren, K. A., & Rojahn, J. (2003). Convergent reliability and validity of the Questions About Behavioral Function and the motivation assessment scale: A replication study. *Journal of Developmental & Physical Disabilities, 15*, 367–375.

Sigafoos, J., Ganz, J. B., O'Reilly, M. F., & Lancioni, G. E. (2008). Evidence-based practice in the classroom: Evaluating a procedure for reducing perseverative requesting in an adolescent with autism and severe intellectual disability. *Australasian Journal of Special Education, 32*, 55–65.

Sigafoos, J., & Meikle, B. (1996). Functional communication training for the treatment of multiply determined challenging behavior in two boys with autism. *Behavior Modification, 20*, 60–84. doi:10.1177/01454455960201003.

Smith, C. M., Smith, R. G., Dracobly, J. D., & Pace, A. P. (2012). Multiple-respondent anecdotal assessments: An analysis of interrater agreement and correspondence with analogue assessment outcomes. *Journal of Applied Behavior Analysis, 45*, 779–795. doi:10.1901/jaba.2012.45-779.

Snell, M. E., Chen, L.-Y., & Hoover, K. (2006). Teaching augmentative and alternative communication to students with severe disabilities: A review of intervention research 1997–2003. *Research & Practice for Persons with Severe Disabilities, 31*, 203–214.

Stokes, T. F., & Osnes, P. G. (1989). An operant pursuit of generalization. *Behavior Therapy, 20*, 337–355.

Volkert, V. M., Lerman, D. C., Call, N. A., & Trosclair-Lasserre, N. (2009). An evaluation of resurgence during treatment with functional communication training. *Journal of Applied Behavior Analysis, 42*, 145–160.

Wacker, D., Lee, J., Padilla Dalmau, Y., Kopelman, T., Lindgren, S., Kuhle, J., …Waldron, D. (2013). Conducting functional communication training via telehealth to reduce the problem behavior of young children with autism. *Journal of Developmental & Physical Disabilities, 25*, 35–48. doi: 10.1007/s10882-012-9314-0.

Walker, V. L., & Snell, M. E. (2013). Effects of augmentative and alternative communication on challenging behavior: A meta-analysis. *Augmentative and Alternative Communication, 29*, 117–131. doi:10.3109/07434618.2013.785020.

Watkins, N., & Rapp, J. T. (2013). The convergent validity of the Questions About Behavioral Function Scale and functional analysis for problem behavior displayed by individuals with autism spectrum disorder. *Research in Developmental Disabilities, 34*, 11–16. doi:10.1016/j.ridd.2012.08.003.

Wilke, A. E., Tarbox, J., Dixon, D. R., Kenzer, A. L., Bishop, M. R., & Kakavand, H. (2012). Indirect functional assessment of stereotypy in children with autism spectrum disorders. *Research in Autism Spectrum Disorders, 6*, 824–828. doi:10.1016/j.rasd.2011.11.003.

Wu, Y., Mirenda, P., Wang, H., & Chen, M. (2010). Assessment and treatment of stereotypic vocalizations in a Taiwanese adolescent with autism: A case study. *International Journal of Special Education, 25*, 160–167.

Zaja, R. H., Moore, L., van Ingen, D. J., & Rojahn, J. (2011). Psychometric comparison of the functional assessment instruments QABF, FACT and FAST for self-injurious, stereotypic and aggressive/destructive behaviour. *Journal of Applied Research in Intellectual Disabilities, 24*, 18–28. doi:10.1111/j.1468–3148.2010.00569.x.

Part III
Controversial Issues in AAC

Chapter 8
The Controversy Surrounding Facilitated Communication

Introduction

Although thoroughly discredited (Mostert 2002), facilitated communication (FC), purportedly a type of augmentative and alternative communication (AAC) that provides a means of communication for individuals who cannot speak, continues to be used and promoted. This chapter provides a description of FC, an overview of the history of the use of FC in the USA, several cautions related to its use, an overview of the research discrediting FC, a discussion of the recent resurgence of FC, and conclusions. Readers are cautioned that this information is provided for informational and cautionary purposes and not as a "how to" description of how to implement FC, which is not recommended.

What Is Facilitated Communication?

FC was developed as a means of providing opportunities for individuals with disabilities that impeded speech, such as autism and cerebral palsy, to communicate via typing or pointing to words or pictures (Crossley 1992). According to the original developers and promoters of FC, the technique involves the following components. One, physical support is provided by a "facilitator," who is an adult who holds or supports the hand of the client (Biklen et al. 1992; Biklen and Schubert 1991). The supposed purpose of this support is to help the client point, but not to make word or letter selections, and provide emotional support. Two, the facilitator provides instruction in FC by asking the client questions and physically prompting the correct answers (Biklen and Schubert 1991). Three, the facilitator assists the client in focusing on the task by redirecting from other activities (such as self-stimulation) through physical and verbal prompts, reminding the client to look at the keyboard, and ignoring echolalia and challenging behaviors (such as pushing the keyboard away; Biklen and Schubert 1991). Four, the facilitator is to avoid testing the client's abilities to correctly answer questions, purportedly to promote the idea that the client is a competent, independent communicator (Biklen and Schubert 1991). Five, the facilitator is to begin "set work," which are tasks that have predictable answers, eventually leading to more open-ended questions (Biklen et al. 1992; Biklen and Schubert 1991). Finally, six, the facilitator is to fade physical support, although Biklen and Schubert (1991) caution that this may take several years.

History of Use of FC

Surprisingly, despite decades of evidence that FC is ineffective and has caused great harm to families (Beck and Pirovano 1996; Hostler et al. 1993; Mostert 2001), FC has been implemented with individuals with CCN since at least the early 1990s. The founders of FC, both in Australia and in the USA, have made a number of claims regarding the efficacy of FC and reasons they believe it cannot be evaluated using traditional scientific methods (Biklen and Schubert 1991; Sheehan and Matuozzi 1996). This history is summarized below.

Founders' Claims

The founders and early adopters of FC have made extraordinary claims regarding skills of individuals, previously unable to communicate, who are suddenly, through FC, found to have previously unimaginable knowledge and skills (Crossley 1992). One such example is a case study of a 7-year old with autism, previously thought of as unable to read or write, who within days of introduction of FC was able to spell multi-syllabic words and, within 2 months, was typing sentences of up to seven words expressing feelings (Biklen and Schubert 1991). An adult with intellectual disabilities who had previously used almost no spontaneous speech and only a few manual signs suddenly began identifying objects correctly and typing complete sentences on the first day she was introduced to FC, though only with physical support (Crossley 1992). A teenage girl who could not speak other than via echolalia reportedly wrote a lengthy, heartfelt letter to her mother (Biklen et al. 1992). Biklen and Schubert (1991) describe case studies of 20 children with autism who, prior to FC, used a few manual signs, had no speech, or had limited speech such as echolalia or simple question-answering were remarkably able to communicate with full sentences with FC implementation; however, in no case did the authors report that physical support had been completely faded for any of the children. One of these children, a 3-year old with autism, surprisingly began to spell words far above the expectations given his age (Biklen and Schubert 1991). A young woman with autism gave a lengthy apology after repeatedly becoming physically aggressive with her facilitator (Biklen et al. 1992). A second-grader reportedly, having never participated in general education instruction, was able to complete complex math problems (Biklen and Schubert 1991). Other remarkable accounts include writing poetry and engaging in lengthy conversation (Biklen and Schubert 1991), skills that are unusual even in individuals with autism who are verbal and high functioning. These claims are not supported by robust research, only case studies (Biklen et al. 1992; Biklen and Schubert 1991; Crossley 1992).

FC proponents have a number of hypotheses to explain why individuals who were previously thought to have little to no language skills and cognitive impairments were suddenly able to demonstrate extraordinary skills and knowledge through FC. These authors suggest that previous conceptualizations of autism, suggesting significant social and language delays, were severely mistaken (Biklen and Schubert 1991) and that when individuals with autism fail to communicate effectively, this is primarily due to anxiety, which can only be addressed through emotional and physical support (Biklen 2003); in other words, through FC. One is the suggestion that, while appearing to avoid others, individuals with autism may be quietly observing and dedicating the brain power that is not used to socialize or speak toward increased intellectual capacity (Biklen and Schubert 1991). Another is the suggestion that, while not appearing to engage in learning activities, these children had learned incidentally via watching their siblings do homework, watching educational television, and while independently leafing through books (Biklen and Schubert 1991). Despite these supposedly marked changes in abilities to understand and use language; apparently many of the individuals using FC continue to engage in challenging behaviors, including aggression, that make their inclusion in community activities difficult (Biklen et al. 1992). This is surprising given that many of these individuals reportedly understood complex language and, presumably, had been told the natural consequences of such behaviors and supposedly had the ability to communicate wants and needs, which typically reduces the need for challenging behavior.

Regarding concerns that typed messages may be initiated by facilitators rather than the clients, the proponents of FC have a number of possible explanations for why they believe this is unlikely (Biklen 2003). One, they claimed that children demonstrated unique phonetic typographical errors in their typing (Biklen and Schubert 1991). Two, they stated that because some of the children required only minimal support, though few have been reported to type independently, it was unlikely that they were being cued (Biklen and Schubert 1991). Three, the children's written words appeared to display unique personalities (Biklen and Schubert 1991). Four, concerns that some children would only "perform" with one facilitator, but not others, are used as opportunities to blame the other potential facilitators for not being supportive of the clients (Biklen and Schubert 1991). Five, Biklen (1996) argues that lack of confidence in the communicative competence of individuals with disabilities leads to poor performance, making controlled studies difficult if not impossible. Six, he also argues that test anxiety resulted in poor performance on tasks in which the facilitators were blind to the questions asked of their clients in controlled studies (Biklen 1995). Such arguments appear to be an attempt to discount any possible means of negating the efficacy of FC. Despite these claims, proponents of FC have been unable to provide convincing evidence that, in most cases, FC is effective and that the messages originate from the individual who has communication needs.

Publications Touting the Reported Benefits of FC

FC has been long debunked (Mostert 2010). However, in the early-to-mid-1990s, a number of articles that appeared to support FC were published in peer-reviewed journals. These were primarily anecdotal or qualitative in nature (e.g., Biklen and Schubert 1991; Broderick and Kasa-Hendrickson 2001; Weiss et al. 1996). One such author (Clarkson 1994) simply extolled the use of FC paired with music therapy, claiming unexpected literacy skills and exploration of feelings as a result of implementation. Another (Olney 1995) provided narrative accounts of FC use in a case study as "evidence," further suggesting that because the individual with autism with whom she worked sometimes typed insults and surprising information, that was indicative of his authorship, despite the author's acknowledgment that she likely led and overinterpreted his communication. Group studies with reportedly positive results had generally poor experimental design. For example, Cardinal et al. (1996) claimed that participants' independent performance had improved when comparing pre–post FC testing; however, they failed to note that neither performances were better than what would be expected by chance. Further, they failed to collect inter-rater reliability data, leaving one to question the validity of their results, and facilitators were never blind to the stimuli presented to the participants, leaving the reader unable to know who authored the messages. Failed attempts to demonstrate consistent patterns of responding were often dismissed with claims that the mechanisms involved in FC are too complex to investigate via traditional scientific procedures and low rates of correct responding in such situations were highlighted as proof, regardless of far higher rates of incorrect responding, the presence of significant redirection and prompting by the facilitators, and lack of inter-rater agreement data (Sheehan and Matuozzi 1996). No well-designed and controlled studies can be found that demonstrate successful use of FC, free from facilitator bias.

Research Negating and Cautions Related to the Dangers of FC

Numerous well-designed studies have made it clear that, in most cases, messages produced via FC are authored by facilitators rather than their clients, or, in some, clients performed better independently than when facilitated (Mostert 2001, 2010). Some of these studies have demonstrated markedly different responses when the facilitator could or could not see the same stimulus as the client (Bebko et al. 1996; Cabay 1994; Hirshoren and Gregory 1995; Kerrin et al. 1998; Montee et al. 1995), poor performance when the facilitator could not see the stimuli or the communication board (Szempruch and Jacobson 1993), and near-chance level responding when the facilitator could not see any stimuli (Regal et al. 1994). Further, researchers (Bebko et al. 1996) demonstrated that most participants performed worse on similar tasks when facilitated but the facilitator could not see the same stimuli compared to their independent performing, suggesting that the use of FC may encourage prompt dependence, or lead to the participants waiting to be prompted instead of attempting independent responding. Additionally, lengthier use of FC appears to correlate with greater degrees of influence of the facilitator on the message produced (Bebko et al. 1996). Studies involved the use of headphones, showing poor performance when the participants and the facilitators heard different words compared to better performance when the participants and facilitators heard the same stimuli (Beck and Pirovano 1996; Hudson et al. 1993). Further, in a study in which the participant and facilitator heard different questions, some of the facilitator's questions were answered correctly, that the participant could not hear, while none of the participant's questions, that the facilitator could not hear, were correct (Hudson et al. 1993). Studies involving facilitators who were blinded to both visual and auditory stimuli found poor performance in participants, even in cases following several months of instruction (Bomba et al. 1996; Eberlin et al. 1993; Smith et al. 1994). Several of the studies indicated that unexpected literacy skills, of the kind suggested by FC proponents (Biklen et al. 1992), were not indicated (Bebko et al. 1996; Eberlin et al. 1993). Some of the studies demonstrating the influence of the facilitator on the message produced using FC implemented multiple methods of evaluation and a range of simple to complex tasks to ensure that results were not due to the designs of the tasks or tasks that were beyond the participants' capabilities, lending more credibility to those studies (e.g., Bebko et al. 1996). Strikingly, some participants whose performances were similar whether or not the facilitator heard or saw the same stimuli or whose performances were poor when the facilitator was blinded were able to independently perform well on the target tasks, via use of AAC (Beck and Pirovano 1996) or manual signs or limited verbalizations (Vázquez 1995).

Proponents of FC have suggested that testing individuals who use FC can cause anxiety, thus suggesting that FC is incompatible with traditional quantitative research methods. Thus, some researchers have designed naturalistic assessments as well, having the participants engage in a leisure or other activity outside of the facilitators' view, then asking questions about the activities (Simon et al. 1994). Such studies demonstrated poor performance on most questions with naïve facilitators and better performance when the facilitators were aware of the activities, indicating a high rate of facilitator leading the answers (Braman et al. 1995; Simon et al. 1994).

Beyond studies evaluating whether the message produced originated from the facilitator or the client with a disability, a series of studies examined the effects of FC on collateral skills and compared the use of FC to other means of communicating. As a result, social interaction and rate of nonfocused interactions (e.g., echolalia or self-stimulatory vocalizations) were not found to improve following FC instruction (Myles et al. 1996a). Further, the combination of direct literacy instruction with FC failed to demonstrate improved phonological and numeracy skills (Myles et al. 1996b). In another study involving reaching comprehension, participants were unable to correctly answer yes/no, multiple choice, and open-ended questions when their facilitators had not read the books themselves, though many could correctly answer questions when their facilitators did know the answers (Simpson and Myles 1995a). When comparing the use of FC to the use of the Picture Exchange Communication System (PECS), Simon et al. (1996) found that a 14-year old who purportedly used FC was unable to correctly identify objects unseen by the facilitator while using FC, was able to correctly and independently identify every object when using PECS.

These studies represent a plethora of attempts to design tasks of various types to provide any possible opportunity to provide evidence for the legitimacy of FC on basic communication skills (e.g., Bebko et al. 1996; Beck and Pirovano 1996; Bomba et al. 1996), academic skills (Myles et al. 1996b), social interaction, and behavior (Myles et al. 1996a). Although some of these studies were case studies (e.g., Simon et al. 1996), the vast majority were well-controlled group studies. All of these studies included at least some participants with ASD. No well-controlled studies with individuals with ASD were able to produce positive results for FC. What is clear is the tendency for well-designed studies to have found FC to be ineffective, while poorly designed studies that lacked controlled procedures (e.g., anecdotal reports, qualitative papers) are those that have claimed positive results (Mostert 2001). Further, the few positive reports (Calculator and Singer 1992) have been criticized (Perry, Bebko, and Bryson 1994) for failing to be replicable; that is, similar studies have failed to have positive findings.

Beyond the lack of evidence establishing FC as an evidence-based practice and evidence demonstrating facilitator leading, there are additional reasons to be cautious in implementation of FC. These cautions relate, primarily, to issues that arise when messages are falsely attributed to the individual with a disability. In the early 1990s, a number of cases involving allegations of child abuse were reported by facilitators whose clients used FC (Hostler et al. 1993). These allegations, in many cases, caused children and adults with developmental disabilities to be taken from their families and placed in protective care, causing skill regression and trauma to the children and their families. Further, in at least one case, failure of the court to validate that the message typed was not led by the facilitator has resulted in a prosecution (Gorman 1999). Hostler et al. (1993) report a number of allegations of sexual abuse were brought in Virginia, noting that in none of the cases were there physical signs of abuse, nor were the patients able to communicate accusations in controlled hospital settings. Similar allegations have been repeatedly falsified through the court and use of simple techniques to test and compare messages typed the facilitators knew the questions asked and when they did not; repeatedly, these tests have indicated that the messages originated from the facilitators (Bligh and Kupperman 1993; Gorman 1999). Additionally, allegations of sexual abuse against parents of two adolescents were dropped following conflicting responses to social questions by two experienced facilitators who were unfamiliar with the adolescents and their cases (Siegel 1995). In combination with the significant evidence that FC messages tend to originate with the facilitator, the repeated false allegations of abuse are a clear signal to avoid use of this means of communication.

Ongoing and Recent Resurgence of Interest in FC

Given the overwhelming evidence that FC is not effective and, in some cases, may cause harm (Mostert 2010), one might question why this topic is still being discussed. Unfortunately, FC and similar methods are still being implemented and promoted in the media and by large and established institutions; sometimes by other names (e.g., Supported Typing, Rapid Prompting) despite the similarities. Although debunked, proponents continue to promote the use of FC and state its efficacy as fact (Mostert 2010). Further, the suggestion that FC cannot be measured via traditional means has been likened to religious beliefs, i.e., faith without proof (Mostert 2010). It is likely that the promulgation of the Internet also allowed FC to be revived because parents of newly diagnosed children who are not aware of over a decade of research debunking FC are unable to differentiate between trustworthy sources of information and are drawn to extraordinary claims, such as those promoted by FC versus other interventions that are more costly in time and money.

The primary promoters of FC are faculty at Syracuse University, where FC had its start in the USA. Despite the evidence of only rare instances in which FC output appeared to be authored by individuals who used AAC (Mostert 2001), and the evidence of numerous false allegations of abuse, these individuals continue to promote the use of FC in the media and through professional publications. In part, they are emphasizing the small number of individuals who appear to, following lengthy implementation of FC, begin typing with little or no physical support (Broderick and Kasa-Hendrickson 2001). The phrase "appear to" is used in this instance because this information comes from promoters of FC via their anecdotal reports or through video that has been significantly edited to prevent the viewer from determining the degree of facilitation. In some cases, individuals who use FC are described as having emerging speech, while still requiring a significant degree of physical support to use FC. For example, Broderick and Kasa-Hendrickson (2001) describe an adolescent, Jamie Burke, who, via FC, would type lengthy, complex conversations, though would speak only by reading what was typed or speaking in short phrases or single words, often prompted, when not relying on typed words. This leads to questions regarding the validity of communications that are only more complex when they have been facilitated. Such stories, such as Jamie Burke's, have been spread via popular magazines as well (Fields-Meyer et al. 2005). Individuals with severe autism, such as Sue Rubin, who has appeared in a documentary and on numerous popular magazine and television reports (e.g., Henneberger 2005), are described going to college, while continuing to have some degree of facilitation. In videos of such individuals, while it is not made clear the degree of facilitation required, there is some visible evidence of prompting; for example, the facilitator is often seated in close physical contact, sometimes holds the keyboard and moves it slightly, and often uses nods and head shakes when the person using FC looks at him or her. These videos suggest subtle cueing develops between the facilitator and the individual with autism. Books purportedly written by a person using FC, Tuomas Alatalo, when examined more closely along with video of him communicating via FC (Saloviita and Sariola 2003; Sturmey 2003), show evidence of discrepancies when different facilitators are used, video in which prerecorded messages were programmed instead of spontaneously typed during interviews, and clips of the facilitators looking intently at the keyboard while Mr. Alatalo looked away at the time he was typing, while there is no evidence of a successful test of authorship or that he could read independently, let alone write.

Conclusions

One might question why facilitators and families become convinced, despite evidence to the contrary, that their clients are suddenly communicating effectively. For one, family members, initially hoping their children will begin to communicate independently, may lose interest in fading prompts as it becomes apparent that the only way their children appear to communicate with great skill is via facilitation, while skills demonstrated independently are inevitably lower level and more simplistic (Sjöholm, and Sjöholm 1994). It may be that, given the rapid appearance of improvement, facilitators themselves begin to believe that their clients are producing the communications (Konstantareas 1998). Further, Simpson and Myles (1995b) reported cases in which facilitators who were found not to have the same level of success with facilitation as other facilitators of the same child were chastised for failing to have faith in the child's ability to communicate or conduction sessions incorrectly. Such peer pressure could lead to inadvertent false positive results.

It is possible that individuals who were originally taught to communicate through facilitation may eventually learn to communicate independently (Biklen 1995). Indeed, Bebko et al. (1996) demonstrated that some individuals who have used FC have been able to perform similarly in independent tasks. However, given that other forms of AAC, such as the PECS and the use of speech-generating devices, have been demonstrated in high-quality studies to have resulted in independent communication (Ganz et al. 2012a, b), it does not seem worth using FC given the risks. Further, if individuals with autism are able to perform independently, it would be prudent to rapidly fade the use of physical supports and prompts, particularly given the evidence that facilitation may sometimes decrease performance if participants become passive in responding (Bebko et al. 1996).

Despite the evidence debunking FC, one might question what harm is done by allowing families to believe that their children, previously thought to have severe disabilities, actually have immense intellectual capacity. The dangers are the same as for the use of or belief in any unproven theory or intervention. For one, resources allocated to FC, such as the salary of a dedicated facilitator, that may be used more efficiently and efficaciously and to provide instruction to the person with autism in effort toward building independence, are instead squandered on a method that requires lifelong dependence. Two, false attribution, such as awarding of unearned degrees and merit, may call to questions all those who have accomplished such achievements honestly, particularly other individuals who use AAC independently. Three, students who used FC for lengthier periods sometimes appeared to perform better during independent tasks than when facilitated (Bebko et al. 1996; Beck and Pirovano 1996), indicating that FC may lead to prompt dependence in individuals who could otherwise communicate independently, lessening the odds that communication that was facilitated was truly indicative of their functioning. Use of FC, if the communication is truly coming from the facilitator, will result in development of an assumed personality that is not based on reality (Levine et al. 1994). Further, that individual's true desires are ignored in this case, in favor of falsely attributed wants (Levine et al. 1994). Four, when a higher level of educational functioning is demonstrated through FC, other necessary and more appropriately leveled functional skills may not be taught, resulting in lack of access to educational opportunities and potentially resulting in significant loss of time and opportunity (Levine et al. 1994).

Understandably, some families may not be convinced until they have tried FC themselves, and unfortunately, their experiences with FC, which often appear to result in discovery of untapped skills and talents, may serve to reinforce the idea that it is effective (Simpson and Myles 1995b). Although not recommended, if practitioners encounter families who believe FC is effective for their children, the following steps are recommended. First, evaluators may test the originality of the message by showing the client an image that the facilitator cannot see and asking questions about the image that cannot be answered without seeing the image (Konstantareas 1998; Shane 1994). Second, facilitation and other physical supports and prompts should be faded rapidly. If the individual is unable to use his or her hands to form a message independently, the practitioner should work with other specialists (e.g., occupational therapists, AAC consultants, speech-language pathologists) to determine whether the problem is physical and requires an adaptation (e.g., head stick pointer) or if the problem is related to cognition (e.g., the individual is not yet reading and requires a drawing or photo-based AAC system). Third, implementers should strongly consider the harm that has resulted from false accusations of abuse when determining whether or not to implement FC and how to communicate to families about FC (Simpson and Myles 1995b). Fourth, one should consider the consequences of implementing FC, such as the resources of time and money that may be better used otherwise to promote learning of functional skills (Simpson and Myles 1995b). In conclusion, although there may appear to be benefits to using FC and situations in which practitioners are required by family members to use FC, it is highly cautioned against and professional ethics typically require practitioners to provide evidence of the efficacy of the interventions they implement, which, in the case of FC, is impossible to provide objectively.

References

Bebko, J. M., Perry, A., & Bryson, S. (1996). Multiple method validation study of facilitated communication: II. Individual differences and subgroup results. *Journal of Autism and Developmental Disorders, 26,* 19–42.

Beck, A. R., & Pirovano, C. M. (1996). Facilitated communicators' performance on a task of receptive language. *Journal of Autism and Developmental Disorders, 26,* 497–512. doi:10.1007/BF02172272.

Bligh, S., & Kupperman, P. (1993). Brief report: Facilitated communication evaluation procedure accepted in a court case. *Journal of Autism and Developmental Disorders, 23,* 553–557.

Biklen, D. (1995). Why parents and children with disabilities should have the right to use facilitated communication. *Exceptional Parent, 25*(7), 48–50.

Biklen, D. (1996). Learning from the experiences of people with disabilities. *American Psychologist, 51,* 985–986. doi:10.1037/0003-066X.51.9.985.

Biklen, D. (2003). Discussion. *Studies in Philosophy & Education, 22,* 371–375.

Biklen, D., Morton, M. W., Gold, D., Berrigan, C., & Swaminathan, S. (1992). Facilitated communication: Implications for individuals with autism. *Topics in Language Disorders, 12*(4), 1–28.

Biklen, D., & Schubert, A. (1991). New words: The communication of students with autism. *Remedial and Special Education, 12*(6), 46–57.

Bomba, C., O'Donnell, L., Markowitz, C., & Holmes, D. L. (1996). Evaluating the impact of facilitated communication on the communicative competence of fourteen students with autism. *Journal of Autism and Developmental Disorders, 26,* 43–58. doi:10.1007/BF02276234.

Braman, B. J., Brady, M. P., Linehan, S. L., & Williams, R. E. (1995). Facilitated communication for children with autism: An examination of face validity. *Behavioral Disorders, 21,* 110–119.

Broderick, A. A., & Kasa-Hendrickson, C. (2001). "Say just one word at first": The emergence of reliable speech in a student labeled with autism. *Journal of the Association for Persons with Severe Handicaps, 26,* 13–24.

Cabay, M. (1994). Brief report: A controlled evaluation of facilitated communication using open-ended and fill-in questions. *Journal of Autism and Developmental Disorders, 24,* 517–527.

Calculator, S. N., & Singer, K. M. (1992). Preliminary validation of facilitated communication. *Topics in Language Disorders, 13,* ix–xvi.

Cardinal, D. N., Hanson, D., & Wakeham, J. (1996). Investigation of authorship in facilitated communication. *Mental Retardation, 34,* 231–242.

Clarkson, G. (1994). Creative music therapy and facilitated communication: New ways of reaching students with autism. *Preventing School Failure, 38,* 31–33.

Crossley, R. (1992). Getting the words out: Case studies in facilitated communication training. *Topics in Language Disorders, 12*(4), 46–59.

Eberlin, M., McConnachie, G., Ibel, S., & Volpe, L. (1993). Facilitated communication: A failure to replicate the phenomenon. *Journal of Autism and Developmental Disorders, 23,* 507–530.

Fields-Meyer, T., Duffy, T., & Arias, R. (2005). Autism: Breaking the silence. *People, 63*(14), 83–86.

Ganz, J. B., Davis, J. L., Lund, E. M., Goodwyn, F. D., & Simpson, R. L. (2012a). Meta-analysis of PECS with individuals with ASD: Investigation of targeted versus non-targeted outcomes, participant characteristics, and implementation phase. *Research in Developmental Disorders, 33,* 406–418. doi:10.1016/j.ridd.2011.09.023.

Ganz, J. B., Earles-Vollrath, T. L., Heath, A. K., Parker, R., Rispoli, M. J., & Duran, J. (2012b). A meta-analysis of single case research studies on aided augmentative and alternative communication systems with individuals with autism spectrum disorders. *Journal of Autism and Developmental Disorders, 42,* 60–74. doi:10.1007/s10803-011-1212-2.

Gorman, B. J. (1999). Facilitated communication: Rejected in science, accepted in court—a case study and analysis of the use of FC evidence under *Frye* and *Daubert. Behavioral Sciences & the Law, 17,* 517–541.

Henneberger, M. (2005). My mind began to wake up. *Newsweek, 145*(9), 52–53.

Hirshoren, A., & Gregory, J. (1995). Further negative findings on facilitated communication. *Psychology in the Schools, 32*, 109–113.

Hostler, S. L., Allaire, J. H., & Christoph, R. A. (1993). Childhood sexual abuse reported by facilitated communication. *Pediatrics, 91*, 1190–1193.

Hudson, A., Melita, B., & Arnold, N. (1993). Brief report: A case study assessing the validity of facilitated communication. *Journal of Autism and Developmental Disorders, 23*, 165–173. doi:10.1007/BF01066425.

Kerrin, R. G., Murdock, J. Y., Sharpton, W. R., & Jones, N. (1998). Who's doing the pointing? Investigating facilitated communication in a classroom setting with students with autism. *Focus on Autism and Other Developmental Disabilities, 13*, 73–79.

Konstantareas, M. M. (1998). Allegations of sexual abuse by nonverbal autistic people via facilitated communication: Testing of validity. *Child Abuse & Neglect, 22*, 1027–1041.

Levine, K., Shane, H. C., & Wharton, R. H. (1994). What if …: A plea to professionals to consider the risk-benefit ratio of facilitated communication. *Mental Retardation, 32*, 300–318.

Montee, B. B., Miltenberger, R. G., & Wittrock, D. (1995). An experimental analysis of facilitated communication. *Journal of Applied Behavior Analysis, 28*, 189–200.

Mostert, M. P. (2001). Facilitated communication since 1995: A review of published studies. *Journal of Autism and Developmental Disorders, 31*, 287–313.

Mostert, M. P. (2002). Letter to the editor: Teaching the illusion of facilitated communication. *Journal of Autism and Developmental Disorders, 32*, 239–240.

Mostert, M. P. (2010). Facilitated communication and its legitimacy—Twenty-first century developments. *Exceptionality, 18*, 31–41.

Myles, B. S., Simpson, R. L., & Smith, S. M. (1996a). Collateral behavioral and social effects of using facilitated communication with individuals with autism. *Focus on Autism and Other Developmental Disabilities, 11*, 163–169.

Myles, B. S., Simpson, R. L., & Smith, S. M. (1996b). Impact of facilitated communication combined with direct instruction on academic performance of individuals with autism. *Focus on Autism and Other Developmental Disabilities, 11*, 37–44.

Olney, M. (1995). Reading between the lines: A case study on facilitated communication. *Journal of the Association for Persons with Severe Handicaps, 20*, 57–65.

Perry, A., Bebko, J. M., & Bryson, S. (1994). Validity of facilitated communication: Failure to replicate Calculator & Singer (1992). *Topics in Language Disorders, 14*, 79–82.

Regal, R. A., Rooney, J. R., & Wandas, T. (1994). Facilitated communication: An experimental evaluation. *Journal of Autism and Developmental Disorders, 24*, 345–355.

Saloviita, T., & Sariola, H. (2003). Authorship in facilitated communication: A re-analysis of a case of assumed representative authentic writing. *Mental Retardation, 41*, 374–379.

Shane, H. (1994). Establishing the source of communication. In H. Shane (Ed.), *Facilitated communication: The clinical and social phenomenon* (pp. 259–299). San Diego CA: Singular Press.

Sheehan, C. M., & Matuozzi, R. T. (1996). Investigation of the validity of facilitated communication through the disclosure of unknown information. *Mental Retardation, 34*, 94–107.

Siegel, B. (1995). Brief report: Assessing allegations of sexual molestation made through facilitated communication. *Journal of Autism and Developmental Disorders, 25*, 319–326. doi:10.1007/BF02179293.

Simon, E. W., Toll, D. M., & Whitehair, P. M. (1994). A naturalistic approach to the validation of facilitated communication. *Journal of Autism and Developmental Disorders, 24*, 647–657.

Simon, E. W., Whitehair, P. M., & Toll, D. M. (1996). A case study: Follow-up assessment of facilitated communication. *Journal of Autism and Developmental Disorders, 26*, 9–18.

Simpson, R. L., & Myles, B. S. (1995a). Effectiveness of facilitated communication with children and youth with autism. *Journal of Special Education, 28*, 424–439.

Simpson, R. L., & Myles, B. S. (1995b). Facilitated communication and children with disabilities: An enigma in search of a perspective. *Focus on Exceptional Children, 27*(9), 1.

Sjöholm, B., & Sjöholm, M. (1994). Facilitated communication and treatment abuse. *Journal of Autism and Developmental Disorders, 24*, 543–549. doi:10.1007/BF02172136.

Smith, M. D., Haas, P. J., & Belcher, R. G. (1994). Facilitated communication: The effects of facilitator knowledge and level of assistance on output. *Journal of Autism and Developmental Disorders, 24*, 357–367.

Sturmey, P. (2003). Typing in tongues: Interesting observations on facilitated communication do not establish authorship. *Mental Retardation, 41*, 386–387.

Szempruch, J., & Jacobson, J. W. (1993). Evaluating facilitated communications of people with developmental disabilities. *Research in Developmental Disabilities, 14*, 253–264.

Vázquez, C. A. (1995). Failure to confirm the word-retrieval problem hypothesis in facilitated communication. *Journal of Autism and Developmental Disorders, 25*, 597–610. doi:10.1007/BF02178190.

Weiss, M. J. S., Wagner, S. H., & Bauman, M. L. (1996). A validated case study of facilitated communication. *Mental Retardation, 34*, 220–230.

Chapter 9
Sign Language Versus Aided AAC

Jennifer B. Ganz and Whitney Gilliland

For several decades, sign language has been promoted as a functional communication option for individuals with ASD who have CCN (Goldstein 2002). The research in support of aided AAC has been highlighted in previous chapters. In this chapter, that support will be compared to the research on the use of sign language as a viable AAC option for individuals with ASD. Further, studies comparing sign language implementation to other communication interventions, including aided AAC, will be reviewed as well as studies investigating the impact of sign language instruction on speech outcomes. The reader is cautioned that this chapter is not intended to promote sign language use with people with ASD. Instead, this information is provided to assist families in making informed choices regarding communication interventions.

Scenario

Jorge was a single father to Max, a 4-year old with autism, who could use a handful of word approximations, primarily in imitation of his father or therapists. Jorge had enrolled Max in an intensive behavioral clinic for a year after learning his diagnosis soon after Max turned 3. Jorge was thrilled with the progress Max was making in preschool skills, behavior, and playing with a larger variety of toys. For one, before beginning therapy, Max would not sit at the table for meals, instead running around the room with his food in hand, coming to the table only to snatch another piece. Jorge was pleased that the therapists had taught him to sit at the table while eating for at least 10 min at a time. However, he was concerned that, although a significant amount of time was spent each week on speech, Max was not improving. He read online about sign language and aided AAC, but both sides claimed theirs was the better option. Jorge wasn't sure whom to believe.

J.B. Ganz, *Aided Augmentative Communication for Individuals with Autism Spectrum Disorders*, Autism and Child Psychopathology Series, DOI 10.1007/978-1-4939-0814-1_9, © Springer Science+Business Media New York 2014

Arguments for the Use of Sign Language with Individuals with ASD

Proponents of sign language have made several arguments for why they believe that sign language is the most appropriate type of AAC for people with ASD. Early reports indicated that although many children with ASD responded to the use of operant conditioning to teach speech, those who were not able to imitate vocalizations often failed to begin to speak (Oxman et al. 1978). Oxman et al. (1978) suggested that children who favor information or stimuli provided through visual means rather than auditory might respond best to sign language instruction. Some argue that manual signs are more transportable; unlike aided AAC, they do not require the "speaker" to bring any equipment, while they always have their hands and, presumably, the ability to use manual signs (Mirenda 2003). Aided AAC equipment may become lost or broken easily and technology may not function as intended (van der Meer et al. 2012c). Further, proponents note that, unlike speech, sign language may be physically prompted; that is, while the mouth cannot be physically manipulated to produce speech through prompting, instructors can use full physical prompts to teach people with ASD to form manual signs (Oxman et al. 1978). The motor skills required for manual signs may be less complex or difficult than those required for speaking (Rotholz et al. 1989). They also argue that many manual signs, unlike spoken language, have a degree of iconicity; that is, the signs often resemble the concepts they impart, while spoken words are abstract and bear no resemblance to the concepts they represent (Oxman et al. 1978; Rotholz et al. 1989). For example, the sign for "cat" in American Sign Language looks as though the speaker is drawing whiskers on his or her face. Many of these arguments, instead of comparing to aided AAC, are based on arguments for why sign language may be a better option than speech instruction for some individuals with ASD.

One the other side, proponents of aided AAC suggest that it is a more appropriate mode of communication for people with ASD and CCN than sign language (Rotholz et al. 1989). For one, aided AAC, like sign language, provides a more concrete and visual symbol representing language concepts than speech; however, aided AAC provides a static symbol, while manual signs are transient. This requires the "listener" to process the symbols in manual signs more rapidly than with AAC symbols and requires the "speaker" to retrieve the vocabulary from his or her long-term memory, versus aided AAC which provides the "speaker" with a menu from which to select (van der Meer et al. 2012a). Not all manual signs are iconic (Rotholz et al. 1989), so they may be too abstract for some people with ASD to comprehend. Considering that many people with ASD also have comorbid ID and that communication impairments are a core characteristic of ASD (APA 2013; Worley and Matson 2012), they may have more difficulty retrieving vocabulary from their memories and using it flexibly and fluently (Mirenda 2003). Finally, fine motor deficits are common in people with ASD (Rotholz et al. 1989; Tincani 2004; van der Meer et al. 2012a), thus making it difficult for them to form intelligible manual signs. All of these issues should certainly be considered when selecting a communication form for an individual with ASD. The evidence behind the communication modes should also be strongly considered.

Research on the Use of Sign Language with People with ASD

Research on the use of sign language with individuals with ASD was first published in the 1970s (see Table 9.1). Several small-scale studies have demonstrated that some individuals with ASD are able to learn to use at least a small number of signs spontaneously and independently (Bonvillian and Nelson 1976; Carr 1979; Hinerman et al. 1982; Remington and Clarke 1983). However, in some cases, the number of vocabulary words was extremely limited or took an inordinate amount of instruction before students could use the signs spontaneously (Carr et al. 1978, 1987; Falcomata et al. 2013; Hinerman et al. 1982; Kee et al. 2012; Remington and Clarke 1983; Valentino and Shillingsburg 2011). In some cases, participants were primarily taught to use signs in highly structured instructional contexts, such as labeling tasks that were then rewarded for correct responses with items that were unrelated (Carr et al. 1978, 1987), rather than natural, functional contexts. In other cases, instructional procedures were not well detailed (Konstantareas et al. 1979; Partington et al. 1994) or involved a wide range of strategies for instruction (Hinerman et al. 1982), including the use of "total communication," or a combination of both sign language and verbal instruction (Konstantareas et al. 1982). Generalization to new contexts and communicative partners and maintenance of skills over time was rarely assessed (see Table 9.1). Further, in many cases, the research designs were weak group designs (Watters et al. 1981) or case studies (Bonvillian and Nelson 1976; Kee et al. 2012; Konstantareas et al. 1982); thus, the literature involving the implementation of manual sign language with people with ASD is difficult to interpret with confidence.

Throughout the research on ASD and manual sign language, it is clear that children with ASD reportedly rarely use sign language spontaneously (Carr and Kologinsky 1983); that is, while they may learn to respond to structured tasks during which signs are elicited, they often do not use these skills in natural contexts. For example, Horner and Budd (1985) found that sign language instruction with an 11-year old with autism in controlled, structured settings did not generalize to natural settings. However, there are a few examples of generalization and flexibility in sign language use in the literature. Carr and Kologinsky (1983) taught three boys with autism, aged 9–14 years, used prompt-fading (from prompts to the presence of the adult) to increase spontaneous signed requests and to promote generalization to new adults. Schepis et al. (1982) provided professional development in naturalistic strategies to promote sign language use to staff members in a residential treatment program for individuals with DD, including four participants with autism. Results indicated increases in the use of unprompted, spontaneous sign language use. In summary, it is a significant problem that much of the research on the use of sign language has investigated labeling tasks that were often reinforced with unrelated items or edibles. It appears that in cases in which participants generalized the use of signs to a variety of context instruction in naturalistic contexts were specifically targeted for intervention (Horner and Budd 1985). Further, in many cases, a small number of signs were acquired by the participants. Thus, little research in this area has demonstrated that sign language instruction has resulted in spontaneous, flexible, functional language use among people with ASD; thus, the purpose of language instruction has not been accomplished via sign language use—at least not as reported in the literature to date.

Table 9.1 Research reporting use of sign language with people with ASD

Author(s)/year	N	Age range (years)	Diagnoses[a]	Participants reported to have some speech[b]	Study design[c]	Communication modality[d]	Maintenance or generalization assessed	Implemented in natural contexts[b,e]	Results
Barrera et al. (1980)	1	4.5	AU	Y	SCD	MS, SC	N	Y	In both groups, percentages for total communication instruction were higher than both oral and sign-alone instructions
Barrera and Sulzer-Azaroff (1983)	3	6–9	AU, DD	Y	SCD	SC, SP	N	N	In all three cases, expressive labels were acquired more quickly in the total communication condition
Bartman and Freeman (2003)	1	2	AU, DD	Y	CS	SC	N	N	The participant appeared to require fewer prompts and begin learning new signs more rapidly throughout the course of the intervention
Beecher and Childre (2012)	3	7–9	AU, DD, ID	Y	SCD-F	MS	N	Y	Two of the three participants improved letter and letter sound knowledge between baseline and intervention; all three improved their sight word knowledge
Bonvillian and Nelson (1976)	1	9	AU	N	CS	MS	N	C	Over a 6-month period, the participant learned to spontaneously use more signs
Brady and Smouse (1978)	1	6	AU	N	SCD	MS, SC, SP	N	N	Vocalization and signing each yielded fewer responses per trial than total communication
Carr et al. (1978)	4	10–15	AU	N	SCD	SC	Y	N	Participants were able to learn to correctly label five objects using signs; skills generalized to additional therapists
Carr and Kologinsky (1983)	6	9–14	AU, ID	N	SCD	MS	Y	N	Participants showed significant improvement in their manual sign language between baseline and intervention
Carr et al. (1987)	4	11–16	AU, DD, SD	N	SCD	MS	Y	N	The participants successfully learned to correctly use up to 45 two-sign phrases to describe what the instructors were doing when asked
Carr et al. (1984)	10	6–11	AU	Y	G	MS, SP	N	N	Children who were initially good verbal imitators demonstrated improved receptive identification in the verbal-only condition; both good and not good imitators did well in the sign language condition

Study	N	Age	Diagnosis		Design	Mode			Outcome
Carbone et al. (2010)	3	4–6	AU, ID	N	SCD	MS	N	N	All participants were able to increase both prompted and unprompted vocalizations in baseline and intervention phases. The number of prompts required also decreased for one participant, while increasing for the other two
Falcomata et al. (2013)	3	2–4	AU, DD	N	SCD	MS	Y	Y (for one participant)	In baseline, participants demonstrated high levels of challenging behavior. During intervention, challenging behavior decreased as requests increased across participants
Fulwiler and Fouts (1976)	1	5	AU	N	CS	MS	Y	N	Although no baseline data were recorded, the participant's use of signed words (cumulative responses) increased significantly from the beginning of the study, over a period of over 20 h
Gregory et al. (2009)	6	7–17	AU, ID	Y	SCD-F	A-AAC; MS	N	Y	Two out of three participants acquired manual sign; however, all three acquired exchange-based communication
Hinerman et al. (1982)	1	5	AU	N	SCD-F	MS	N	N	The participant was able to meet criteria across all three conditions
Horner and Budd (1985)	1	11	AU, ID	Y	SCD-F	MS	Y	Y	Participant was able to meet criteria in simulation training for all five signs. The participant was also able to sign all five signs in the natural setting
Kee et al. (2012)	1	28	AU, DD, SD	N	SCD-F	MS	Y	Y	The mean requesting for "eat" increased significantly between baseline and intervention for "eat"; however, there was no improvement in the participant's use of the sign "drink" between baseline and intervention
Konstantareas et al. (1979)	4	8–10	AU, ID	Y	SCD-F	SC	N	N	Each individual acquired new signs, including spontaneous signs
Konstantareas et al. (1982)	1	10	AU, DD, SD	Y	CS	MS, SC	N	NS	Authors report that participants gained 26 signs
Konstantareas and Leibovitz (1981)	8	5–11	AU, ID	N	G	MS, SC	N	N	Simultaneous communication appeared to result in better receptive and expressive language gains when compared with signing plus nonverbally mouthing words

(continued)

Table 9.1 (continued)

Author(s)/year	N	Age range (years)	Diagnoses[a]	Participants reported to have some speech[b]	Study design[c]	Communication modality[d]	Maintenance or generalization assessed	Implemented in natural contexts[b,e]	Results
Kouri (1988)	5	2–4	AU, ID; OTH	N	SCD	MS	N	N	The one participant who had autism did appear to improve in use of sign language and spontaneous words; however, there was not a clear functional relation between the intervention and the outcome variables
Partington et al. (1994)	1	6	AU	N	SCD-F	MS	N	Y	The participant learned more signs to label when nonverbal stimuli were introduced and verbal prompts were reduced
Remington and Clarke (1983)	2	10–15	AU	One nonverbal, other verbal	SCD	MS, SC	N	N	The participants learned to label via sign with both manual sign-alone and simultaneous communication instructions
Rotholz et al. (1989)	2	17–18	AU	N	SCD	A-AAC, MS	Y	Y	Communication book instruction resulted in a higher percentage of understandable communication than sign language. Communication book accuracy was also high
Salvin et al. (1977)	1	5	AU	N	CS	MS	N	C	Participant was able to increase expressive signs, but did not increase verbal communication
Schaeffer et al. (1977)	3	4–5	AU	N	CS	MS, SC	NS	N	Over a 3-year period, all participants made improvements in sign language and developed some spontaneous speech
Schepis et al. (1982)	5	18–21	AU, ID	Y	SCD	MS, SC	N	N	Averages increased between baseline and intervention for signing. Total signing was more effective than nonphysically prompted signing
Tincani (2004)	2	5–6	AU, ID	N	SCD	A-AAC, MS	N	Y	Participants varied with regard to which communication mode they performed best
Valentino and Shillingsburg (2011)	1	7	AU	N	SCD	SC	N	N	The participant increased sign language requesting, labeling, and responding to verbal cues more often after sign language exposure

Study	N	Age	Diagnosis		Design	Intervention			Results
van der Meer et al. (2012a)	4	6–13	AU, ID, PDD	Y	SCD	A-AAC, MS	Y	N	All participants met mastery criteria for aided AAC, while only half met criteria for sign language. The two participants who made it to follow-up chose to use an SGD over all other interventions
van der Meer et al. (2012b)	4	5–10	AU, DD	Y	SCD	A-AAC, MS	Y	Y	Three of the four participants mastered use of manual signs, while all mastered use of an SGD. Three individuals preferred SGD over MS during follow-up. One individual chose MS on over half of sessions
van der Meer et al. (2012c)	4	4–11	AU, DD, ID	Y	SCD	A-AAC, MS	Y	Y	Three of the four students chose the SGD over manual signs during the follow-up trials. Three of the students also performed better using the speech-generating device
Walker et al. (1982)	1	5	AU	Y	SCD-F	MS	Y	N	The individual showed a significant increase in the percentage of signs between baseline and generalization. No data were reported during the intervention
Watters et al. (1981)	4	10–16	AU, DD	N	CS	SC	N	Y	Participants were taught four receptive and expressive signs. They appeared to learn more quickly when expressive was taught before receptive than vice versa
Wherry and Edwards (1983)	1	5	AU	Y	SCD	MS, SC	N	N	The cumulative number correct was the most for signs and the least for verbal, with simultaneous communication in the middle. Subject-initiated interactions varied significantly in verbal and physical interactions, as well as eye contact
Yoder and Layton (1988)	60	2–5	AU	Y	G	MS, SC, SP	N	N	The difference between speech-alone, simultaneous communication and alternating presentation of sign and speech was small

[a]AU autism, autistic disorder, early infantile autism, DD developmental delay, developmental disability, ID intellectual disability, mental retardation, PDD pervasive developmental disorder, not otherwise specified, SD sensory disability, OTH other disabilities (e.g., chromosomal abnormalities); diagnosis definitions listed here reflect the terms used in the original articles, though they may be outdated. All participants are included in the study N; In some cases, some participants had ASD while others had other DD or ID

[b]NS not stated in the article

[c]CS case study, narrative description (interpret results with caution), G group study, SCD robust single-case design, SCD-F single-case design with significant design flaws (interpret results with caution)

[d]A-AAC aided AAC, MS manual sign language, SC simultaneous communication (speech and sign language implemented together), SP speech

[e]C combination of instruction in both natural and analogue contexts

Assertions Regarding the Use of Sign Language to Promote Speech Acquisition

Assertions that instruction in manual sign language would promote speech in people with ASD were made as early as the 1970s (Carr 1979). Unfortunately, it appears that most of these studies were presented at professional conferences and were not published in peer-reviewed journal articles, thus making it difficult to access that information. At that time, it was noted that only some, but not all, children's speech improved following sign language instruction, though most did appear to be able to learn some sign language. Further, Carr (1979) suggested that children who demonstrate some echolalia or verbal imitation skills are more likely to begin speaking when sign language instruction (simultaneous communication training, or the use of both speech and sign language models) occurs than those who do not initially use any words. In the 1970s sign language proponents suggested that simultaneous communication training, also referred to as signed speech plus total communication training, was more likely to result in spontaneous, flexible speech than traditional, discrete trial format speech instruction (Schaeffer et al. 1977). Early proponents of simultaneous communication suggested that sign language might provide a visual support to learning auditory information (Konstantareas and Leibovitz 1981), given that people with autism generally have poor receptive language skills compared to the general population (APA 2013). They further suggested that sign language may allow for easier processing than verbal language, given that it may be spoken more slowly, and that instructors are able to provide physical prompts, which is not possible with speech instruction (Konstantareas and Leibovitz 1981).

Early reports of sign language stimulating speech were primarily in the form of case studies reporting results much after treatment began (Fulwiler and Fouts 1976; Schaeffer et al. 1977). That is, it is difficult to determine from these reports the exact nature of the treatment and whether or not there were other factors that may have contributed to the development of language in these children or whether they would have begun to speak regardless of sign language intervention. Other studies in the 1970s included group studies with groups so small (e.g., four participants) that is difficult to generalize to larger populations (Konstantareas and Leibovitz 1981). A small number of more recent studies have reported positive results related to speech after simultaneous communication instruction (Barrera and Sulzer-Azaroff 1983; Carbone et al. 2010; Valentino et al. 2012). In many cases, the studies involved highly structured activities in highly contrived contexts (Valentino et al. 2012), and spontaneous, functional speech was not reported (Carbone et al. 2010; Konstantareas and Leibovitz 1981). In some of this research, participants already had some speech, such as immediate echolalia (Barrera and Sulzer-Azaroff 1983), making it difficult to generalize these results to people with ASD who have no prior speech abilities. In one case, the author has a significant conflict of interest (Carbone et al. 2010); that is, he is the director of a clinic that specializes in this method and presents these methods widely.

In a few cases, studies have reported mixed results or no impact on speech. For example, four elementary-aged children were taught using simultaneous communication over 9 months (Konstantareas et al. 1979), resulting in improvements in sign language use in imitation, receptive answering of questions, and spontaneous use. Two of the children began using some speech, though the other two did not. Procedures included implementation during naturalistic activities, modeling of signs, and simultaneous use of manual signs and speech by the teachers; however, few details are provided. Salvin et al. (1977) reported on a case study with a 5-year old with autism and ID who was able to learn 12 manual signs over a 3-month instructional period. The researchers reported no improvements in speech use.

Research on the Impact of Sign Language Instruction on Challenging Behaviors

A small number of studies have reported that problem behaviors were reduced as a result of sign language instruction. Horner and Budd (1985) implemented sign language instruction with an 11-year old with autism, finding that naturalistic sign language instruction resulted in a reduction in problem behaviors. Kee et al. (2012) noted anecdotally that the adult they taught to use two signs displayed fewer instances of escape behavior as a result of intervention. Further, functional communication training (discussed in further detail in Chap. 7) involves conducting a functional analysis, or manipulation of conditions to determine why the child is engaging in challenging behaviors (Mancil 2006), and teaching a more socially appropriate means of communication. In some cases, manual sign language may be used (Falcomata et al. 2013) if the participant is unable to speak effectively. Falcomata et al. (2013) implemented FCT using a combination of a picture-selection AAC system, which was faded and replaced with sign language approximations, in a multiple baseline design with three participants, two of whom had autism. Their findings indicated that the participants learned at least two sign approximations and challenging behaviors decreased. No other studies involving the implementation of sign language as a component of FCT for individuals with ASD have been published to date. There is not a large base of research supporting the use of manual sign language to reduce problem behaviors in people with ASD and CCN.

Comparisons Between Sign Language and Other Language Instruction

Most comparisons between sign language instruction and instruction in other language modalities, such as speech or aided AAC, have taken place recently. Simultaneous communication was found to have better impacts than sign language-alone and speech-only on receptive language (Brady and Smouse 1978). Others found little difference in outcomes when comparing sign, speech, and simultaneous communication (Wherry and Edwards 1983). When sign language instructions has been compared to aided AAC, results have varied. In many cases, some participants performed better with sign language while others performed better with aided AAC (Tincani 2004; van der Meer et al. 2012a, b), participants performed equally well in different conditions (Gregory et al. 2009), or participants performed better in aided AAC conditions than in sign language conditions (van der Meer et al. 2012c). Several of the abovementioned studies were limited by small numbers of participants, small numbers of vocabulary words taught (Brady and Smouse 1978), a lack of baseline data via which to compare intervention performance, a lack of generalization and maintenance data (Gregory et al. 2009), and the use of highly controlled versus naturalistic procedures (Carr et al. 1984; Wherry and Edwards 1983). Preference has been investigated in a few studies that included comparisons between sign language and aided AAC. In those studies, results related to preference were generally mixed and there was not a clear connection between preference and performance for all participants (van der Meer et al. 2012a, b). One robust research design involved random assignment of 60 children with ASD to four treatment groups, speech-only, sign-only, simultaneous communication, and alternation between the other three treatments (Yoder and Layton 1988). Findings indicated that pretreatment verbal imitation skills, not treatment conditions, were predictive of growth in speech in the participants. Although other works have been cited in support of the use of manual sign language over selection-based, aided AAC (e.g., Sundberg and Sundberg 1990; Wraikat et al. 1991), these works were conducted with individuals with DD who did not have ASD and, thus, are not included in this review.

Conclusions

Clearly, more research is needed on the role of preference and participant characteristics related to AAC modality, and substantive statements related to the use of sign language versus aided AAC cannot be made. It appears to be likely that the selected language intervention should be tailored to the individual characteristics of the child. The necessity to match learner characteristics to selected communications systems was stated as early as the 1970s (Bonvillian and Nelson 1976). This points to the need for larger scale investigations comparing the use of sign language and aided AAC systems, either via randomized controlled trials or meta-analysis of single-case research. Further, it is critical that researchers include measures of cognitive functioning, severity of ASD symptoms, and verbal imitation skills to enable the determination of efficacy of each type of AAC differentiated by participant characteristics.

References

American Psychiatric Association [APA]. (2013). *Diagnostic and statistical manual* (5th ed.). Washington, DC: Author.

Barrera, R. D., Lobato-Barrera, D., & Sulzer-Azaroff, B. (1980). A simultaneous treatment comparison of three expressive language training programs with a mute autistic child. *Journal of Autism and Developmental Disorders, 10,* 21–37.

Barrera, R., & Sulzer-Azaroff, B. (1983). An alternating treatment comparison of oral and total communication training programs with echolalic autistic children. *Journal of Applied Behavior Analysis, 16,* 379–394.

Bartman, S., & Freeman, N. (2003). Teaching language to a two-year-old with autism. *Journal of Developmental Disabilities, 10,* 47–53.

Beecher, L., & Childre, A. (2012). Increasing literacy skills for students with intellectual and developmental disabilities: Comprehensive reading instruction with sign language. *Education and Training in Autism and Developmental Disabilities, 47*, 487–501.

Bonvillian, J. D., & Nelson, K. E. (1976). Sign language acquisition in a mute autistic boy. *Journal of Speech and Hearing Disorders, 41*, 339–347.

Brady, D. O., & Smouse, A. D. (1978). A simultaneous comparison of three methods for language training with an autistic child: An experimental single case analysis. *Journal of Autism and Childhood Schizophrenia, 8*, 271–279.

Carbone, V. J., Sweeney-Kerwin, E., Attanasio, V., & Kasper, T. (2010). Increasing the vocal responses of children with autism and developmental disabilities using manual sign mand training and prompt delay. *Journal of Applied Behavior Analysis, 43*, 705–709.

Carr, E. G. (1979). Teaching autistic children to use sign language: Some research issues. *Journal of Autism and Developmental Disorders, 9*, 345–359.

Carr, E. G., Binkoff, J. A., Kologinsky, E., & Eddy, M. (1978). Acquisition of sign language by autistic children. I: Expressive labelling. *Journal of Applied Behavior Analysis, 11*, 489–501.

Carr, E. G., & Kologinsky, E. (1983). Acquisition of sign language by autistic children II: Spontaneity and generalization effects. *Journal of Applied Behavior Analysis, 16*, 297–314. doi:10.1901/jaba.1983.16-297.

Carr, E. G., Kologinsky, E., & Leff-Simon, S. (1987). Acquisition of sign language by autistic children. III: Generalized descriptive phrases. *Journal of Autism & Developmental Disorders, 17*, 217–229. doi:10.1007/BF01495057.

Carr, E. G., Pridal, C., & Dores, P. A. (1984). Speech versus sign comprehension in autistic children: Analysis and prediction. *Journal of Experimental Child Psychology, 37*, 587–597.

Falcomata, T. S., Wacker, D. P., Ringdahl, J. E., Vinquist, K., & Dutt, A. (2013). An evaluation of generalization of mands during functional communication training. *Journal of Applied Behavior Analysis, 46*, 444–454. doi:10.1002/jaba.37.

Fulwiler, R. L., & Fouts, R. S. (1976). Acquisition of American sign language by a noncommunicating autistic child. *Journal of Autism and Childhood Schizophrenia, 6*, 43–51.

Goldstein, H. (2002). Communication intervention for children with autism: A review of treatment efficacy. *Journal of Autism & Developmental Disorders, 32*, 373–396.

Gregory, M. K., DeLeon, I. G., & Richman, D. M. (2009). The influence of matching and motor-imitation abilities on rapid acquisition of manual signs and exchange-based communicative responses. *Journal of Applied Behavior Analysis, 42*, 399–404. doi:10.1901/jaba.2009.42-399.

Hinerman, P. S., Jenson, W. R., Walker, G. R., & Petersen, P. B. (1982). Positive practice overcorrection combined with additional procedures to teach signed words to an autistic child. *Journal of Autism and Developmental Disorders, 12*, 253–263.

Horner, R. H., & Budd, C. (1985). Acquisition of manual sign use: Collateral reduction of maladaptive behavior, and factors limiting generalization. *Education and Training of the Mentally Retarded, 20*, 39–47.

Kee, S. B., Casey, L. B., Cea, C. R., Bicard, D. F., & Bicard, S. E. (2012). Increasing communication skills: A case study of a man with autism spectrum disorder and vision loss. *Journal of Visual Impairment & Blindness, 106*, 120–125.

Konstantareas, M. M., Hunter, D., & Sloman, L. (1982). Training a blind autistic child to communicate through signs. *Journal of Autism and Developmental Disorders, 12*, 1–11.

Konstantareas, M. M., & Leibovitz, S. F. (1981). Early communication acquisition by autistic children: Signing & mouthing vs. signing & speaking. *Sign Language Studies, 31*, 135–154.

Konstantareas, M. M., Webster, C. D., & Oxman, J. (1979). Manual language acquisition and its influence on other areas of functioning in four autistic and autistic-like children. *Journal of Child Psychology and Psychiatry, and Allied Disciplines, 20*, 337–350.

Kouri, T. A. (1988). Effects of simultaneous communication in a child-directed treatment approach with preschoolers with severe disabilities. *Augmentative and Alternative Communication, 4*, 222–232.

Mancil, G. R. (2006). Functional communication training: A review of the literature related to children with autism. *Education & Training in Developmental Disabilities, 41*, 213–224.

Mirenda, P. (2003). Toward functional augmentative and alternative communication for students with autism: Manual signs, graphic symbols, and voice output communication aids. *Language, Speech, and Hearing Services in Schools, 34*, 203–216.

Oxman, J., Webster, C. C., & Konstantareas, M. M. (1978). The perception and processing of information by severely dysfunctional nonverbal children: A rationale for the use of manual communication. *Sign Language Studies, 21*, 289–316.

Partington, J. W., Sundberg, M. L., Newhouse, L., & Spengler, S. M. (1994). Overcoming an autistic child's failure to acquire a tact repertoire. *Journal of Applied Behavior Analysis, 27*, 733–734.

Remington, B., & Clarke, S. (1983). Acquisition of expressive signing by autistic children: An evaluation of the relative effects of simultaneous communication and sign-alone training. *Journal of Applied Behavior Analysis, 16*, 315–328.

Rotholz, D. A., Berkowitz, S. F., & Burberry, J. (1989). Functionality of two modes of communication in the community by students with developmental disabilities: A comparison of signing and communication books. *The Journal of the Association for Persons with Severe Handicaps, 14*, 227–233.

Salvin, A., Routh, D. K., Foster, R. E., & Lovejoy, K. M. (1977). Acquisition of modified American sign language by a mute autistic child. *Journal of Autism and Childhood Schizophrenia, 7*, 359–371.

Schaeffer, B., Killinzas, G., Musil, A., & McDowell, P. (1977). Spontaneous verbal language for autistic children through signed speech. *Sign Language Studies, 17*, 287–328.

Schepis, M., Reid, D., Fitzgerald, J. R., Faw, G., Pol, R., & Welty, P. (1982). A program for increasing manual signing by autistic and profoundly retarded youth within the daily environment. *Journal of Applied Behavior Analysis, 15*, 363–379.

Sundberg, C. T., & Sundberg, M. L. (1990). Comparing topography-based verbal behavior with stimulus selection-based verbal behavior. The Analysis of Verbal Behavior, *8*, 83–99.

Tincani, M. (2004). Comparing the picture exchange communication system and sign language training for children with autism. *Focus on Autism & Other Developmental Disabilities, 19*, 152–163.

Valentino, A. L., & Shillingsburg, M. A. (2011). Acquisition of mands, tacts, and intraverbals through sign exposure in an individual with autism. *Analysis of Verbal Behavior, 27*, 95–101.

Valentino, A. L., Shillingsberg, M. A., & Call, N. A. (2012). Comparing the effects of echoic prompts and echoic prompts plus modeled prompts on intraverbal behavior. *Journal of Applied Behavior Analysis, 45*, 431–435.

van der Meer, L., Didden, R., Sutherland, D., O'Reilly, M., Lancioni, G., & Sigafoos, J. (2012a). Comparing three augmentative and alternative communication modes for children with developmental disabilities. *Journal of Developmental and Physical Disabilities, 24*, 451–468. doi:10.1007/s10882-012-9283-3.

van der Meer, L., Kagohara, D., Achmadi, D., O'Reilly, M., Lancioni, G., Sutherland, D., & Sigafoos, J. (2012b). Speech-generating devices versus manual signing for children with developmental disabilities. *Research in Developmental Disabilities, 33*, 1658–1669.

van der Meer, L., Sutherland, D., O'Reilly, M. F., Lancioni, G. E., & Sigafoos, J. (2012c). A further comparison of manual signing, picture exchange, and speech-generating devices as communication modes for children with autism spectrum disorders. *Research in Autism Spectrum Disorders, 6*, 1247–1257.

Walker, G. R., Hinerman, P. S., Jenson, W. R., & Peterson, P. B. (1982). Sign language as a prompt to teach a verbal "yes" and "no" discrimination to an autistic boy. *Child and Family Behavior Therapy, 3*, 77–86.

Watters, R., Wheeler, L., & Watters, W. (1981). The relative efficiency of two orders for training autistic children in the expressive and receptive use of manual signs. *Journal of Communication Disorders, 14*, 273–285.

Wherry, J. N., & Edwards, R. P. (1983). A comparison of verbal, sign, and simultaneous systems for the acquisition of receptive language by an autistic boy. *Journal of Communication Disorders, 16*, 201–216.

Worley, J. A., & Matson, J. L. (2012). Comparing symptoms of autism spectrum disorders using the current "DSM-IV-TR" diagnostic criteria and the proposed "DSM-V" diagnostic criteria. *Research in Autism Spectrum Disorders, 6*, 965–970.

Wraikat, R., Sundberg, C., & Michael, J. (1991). Topography-based and selection-based verbal behavior: A further comparison. The Analysis of Verbal Behavior, *9*, 1–17.

Yoder, P. J., & Layton, T. L. (1988). Speech following sign language training in autistic children with minimal verbal language. *Journal of Autism and Developmental Disorders, 18*, 217–229.

Index